I'M NOT GLOWING, I'M GOING TO POKE YOU IN THE EYE

SURVIVING PREGNANCY SURPRISES – WHAT THEY DON'T TELL YOU TO EXPECT

V. PAUL

I dedicate this book to my family - with special thanks to my mom and sister who catered to my every whim during my pregnancy. I also dedicate this book to my late father, who left us too soon - some day our souls will meet again.

DISCLAIMER

First Trimester

I KNEW WITHIN FOUR WEEKS OF CONCEPTION THAT I WAS PREGNANT.

Bleh, *I feel pregnant*, I thought to myself absentmindedly one morning, as I was making my coffee. The idea got more concrete in my head as I contemplated it some more throughout the day. This was a huge surprise to me, since I had never been pregnant before. I always had highly irregular periods, so I couldn't tell if I was late or missing a period.

I did always felt a bit queasy about a week before my period showed up, but this time I felt that nauseous feeling for four weeks straight, and I also had a new symptom - sore boobs for an equal length of time. I vaguely remembered having read something somewhere about pregnancy symptoms and asked my surprised hubby to pick up a test on his way home from work.

"A what?" hubby asked without much surprise in

his voice that I could discern over the phone, probably sure that he had misheard me.

"Could you pick up a pregnancy test thingamajigger." I repeated, stirring the chicken in the saucepan.

"Oh. Are you sure?" he sounded a little surprised now.

"Obviously not, honey, or I wouldn't need a test to find out. It's probably nothing. I mean, there's no way possible I could be pregnant... we were fairly careful. Weren't we?"

"Ah." he paused, "A couple of nights, we weren't really."

"There's no way a couple of nights of not being careful would end up with me getting pregnant. *Definitely not*. That'd be nothing short of miraculous." I scoffed. "But I just want to be sure, just in case there's the .000001 percent chance that I am."

"So... what kind?"

"I have no idea. Just pick something, your guess is as good as mine." I responded.

"Alright, hun," he sounded pretty normal, surprisingly. Then again, I have no idea what the expression on his face may have been as he hung up the phone.

Ah yes, the hubby. He had wanted to wait at least a year or two after marriage before having kids. We were three months into our marriage when this telephone conversation happened, the day before hubby's birthday, in late January.

My husband and I had finally agreed at the beginning of the year, that we would try to have a baby starting around May. This had been a point of conflict for us both for a while - we had just married each other the past November, and he wanted to enjoy some time by ourselves as a married couple for a few years before we had kids. I, on the other hand, being two years older than him, at 33 years old (turning 34 the upcoming May), was eager to start our family sooner. We fought, we argued, we cried. Okay - only I cried, and mostly when no one was looking.

The first order of business the week after we got married was to add a furry member to our family - and so we were already a family of three. We got a spunky, stubborn German Shepherd puppy. Hubby was not at all fond of dogs at the time, but he welcomed the furry little girl with open arms. She definitely tested his patience and he had to compromise on his almost OCD need to keep things exceptionally clean and organized - he almost couldn't handle it when she had the to-be-expected puppyhood accidental pees and poos on the living room floor. It drove him nuts when she chewed up all her doggy toys and scattered them all over the place. He almost lost his mind when she ate the wooden kitchen chair leg. The first time he had to clean up an accident of puppy poop from the floor, he nearly vomited.

"It's good practice for you," I had smiled, "for when you have to change baby diapers. And you need to get rid of a mess, trust me, when we have kids, there will be toys everywhereeeee"

"Not for a long while!" he'd quip back, ignoring my pout. "And besides, you can train kids to put things back in their place on shelves."

"Yeah, you're in some sort of fantasy world if you think the house is always going to be clean once kids arrive."

"Mitt's kids put everything back in place once they're done playing." he said matter of factly.

"Mitt's kids are 5 and 7 years old, aren't they? And you think they're going to have visitors over without cleaning their house? How do you know what it looks like on an off-day?" I questioned, very amused at his complete ignorance of what it must be like to have your own kids at home, whilst also wondering if it would indeed be possible for such a feat to be accomplished. "They probably had their own share of crayoned walls and spills to clean."

"All I'm saying is that their house is always perfectly organized and clean and they have two kids." he said.

I laughed out loud. "Oh man, you really do believe that, don't you?" knowing at that moment that having a puppy would be the absolute best intro for him to get a taste of what it would be like to take care of a child. It made me also realize that perhaps it would be a good idea to wait a while before having a child of our own so he could get acclimated to taking care of a furry-baby - if he was unable to handle the smaller messes that a puppy made, he would be overwhelmed with the giant messes a toddler would eventually make. I had always noted that he liked everything to be a certain way, and had a very low tolerance level for disorganization. It was a wonderful attribute to have, since I, on the other hand, was the type of person who had an "organized mess" lifestyle. It helped me learn to become a bit more organized and I was able to appreciate the value in being more structured. I'd try my hardest to keep things somewhat tidy, and he'd try to overlook the 'mess' I created, as he called it - in other words, a small pile of clothes in one corner of our room, or items I'd shove into the kitchen drawer that were supposed to go into a different drawer. It still didn't prepare him for having a puppy.

During the first couple of months that we had her, he'd constantly be walking around like a zombie saying, "We need to drop the stress level here with her."

I'd be baffled, and ask, "What stress? I'm not stressed about her. She's still learning. She's actually a great dog, and super smart! It takes about 6 months for a dog to be fully house trained, you know."

It would irritate me that he couldn't get past this, and occasionally it would blow up into huge fights between us as I questioned his inability to deal with what I believed was a regular part of dog ownership. "If you can't look after one little dog, how can you ever look after a child?!"

"A dog is not the same as a child!" he'd snip back. "And a child won't poop on the floor constantly since they have diapers!"

In fairness to him, when I think about it now, he had never owned a dog of his own before and he had no idea how to train one. I had a few dogs while growing up and much more experience with training and expectations. I knew there'd be a rainbow after the rain, and that it would just be a few more months till she was house-broken. In his mind, he couldn't see how the accidents would ever stop if they hadn't already. It didn't help that we lived on a split-level condo that we had to go down to the first floor to let her out. The living room was on the second floor and by the time the little puppy realized she had to go out, she'd only make it to the stairs before peeing all over the carpet on her way down. She was unable to reach the front door in time to let us know she had to go out. Eventually she gave up and just peed where she stood.

One evening, after she had soiled the floor yet again without letting out so much as a whimper or a bark to tell us, he pleaded, "Can't you train her to tell us properly when she needs to go out? A friend of mine said you can train a dog to ring a bell to go out."

"What? That's amazing!" I exclaimed, and got to work researching it online. I'd never heard of that before and didn't fully believe it was possible, but doggone it, I was going to try.

I bought her a Poochie-Bell door-strap from Amazon that had great reviews, and started training her. Hubby had installed a baby gate at the top of the stairs and I hung the bells on it. In less than two days, she had mastered the concept and was pawing at the bells to be let out. I was so pleased by this that I made a tutorial video and posted it on YouTube. Most importantly, it wasn't until I had trained her to do this that Hubby's stress level dipped considerably. No more pee in the house, woohoo!

Over several months, he learned to cope with the rest of it. He still hated when she left her dog toys out, but would just kick them out of his path rather than letting his head explode. When she scratched up our wooden front door one day, he just shook his head and said "What did you do? Look at what she did!" before grabbing her and rubbing her head affectionately. She wagged her tail happily. He wasn't pleased, but he was less reactive to it. Or maybe his growing love for her just made it easier for him to overlook her misbehavior. He had really grown fond of her, and was constantly amazed at her intelligence and personality. He had always just looked at a dog as a furry ball of drool, but she earned his love with her devotion. Doggy and Hubby were soon best of friends, even after she ate three pairs of his expensive leather shoes. I was ecstatic. It gave me the warm and fuzzies to watch them bond. My heart was especially warmed one night when he found a blankie to put over her and actually tucked her in for bedtime.

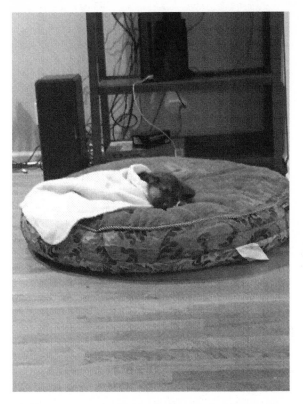

Hubby eventually gave in and withdrew his "after a few years" schedule before we started trying to have a human kid of our own, making it "after a few months" because I also had concerns about turning 35 and being considered a 'high risk' or 'geriatric pregnancy' due to my age alone. I was also worried that I would not be able to conceive right away since almost a third of my friends and various other people I knew of had trouble conceiving or else needed fertility treatments. I fully expected that it would take at least a year of trying before I got pregnant. Especially since I was so irregular as well. So, we weren't really 'meticulously careful', although we did try to be 'careful' and figured if I got pregnant, then I did. In hindsight, he was right - our marriage could have used that year of bliss - having a baby changed everything, but that's a story for another day.

As it turned out, three months after we got married, there I was standing in the washroom, staring at a pregnancy stick.

2

So, there are two lines that you have to look out for when taking your standard off-the-shelf pregnancy test. My husband came home with the First Response brand. One line always appears - it shows up immediately after you pee on it. Apparently, this test line is there to make sure that it is a working testing stick. The other line either shows up or it doesn't. If it shows up, you're pregnant. Right? Not quite.

I always thought (having never taken a pregnancy test before) that the single dark line suggested a negative result and two very visible lines suggested a positive result. Nobody ever mentioned the possibility of a very faint, barely-there line. When Hubby got home, we both just looked at each other without saying much. There was an air of excitement between us, it was like we both wanted to know and yet didn't want to know. He handed the pregnancy test box to me and I ripped open the package and headed to the washroom.

"Well?!" Hubby called out a minute later as he stood outside the door.

"I'm reading the instructions!" I called back. The instructions were fairly simple. In the results section, it stated the following:

"PREGNANT: Two Pink Lines appear in the Easy Read Result Window. Note: One line may be lighter than the other. NOT PREGNANT: Only One Pink Line appears in the Easy Read Result Window."

I took a deep breath and then peed on that little stick. An extremely faint line gradually appeared on my home pregnancy test as I stared at it, waiting for the required number of minutes – but it was hardly visible. I waited for it to get darker, but it didn't. It was so faint that I wasn't sure if I was just seeing things. There was also the very dark pink line as well, that showed up immediately. I squinted in confusion. I couldn't believe it. I had to look at it really, really, closely because the line was barely there. But it was there. Wasn't this supposed to be a life-changing moment? The moment I knew for sure and jumped up and down screaming with joy? I stared silently at the stick for quite a while before coming out of the washroom to let my husband know the results.

"Well?" he asked softly and curiously, obviously noting the expression on my face.

"Um… I'm not sure." was my answer. He was expecting a "yes" or "no" answer too, it turned out.

I spent the next five hours on my computer and iPhone searching on google for "pregnancy test results, faint pink line, barely visible" with several variations in wording. They all said it would be best to test first thing in the morning when your pee is most concentrated and the pregnancy hormone would have a stronger presence. So, I tested it again the next morning. Sure enough, the second line showed up again. A little stronger, but still quite faint. This, according to omnipotent and all-knowing Google, was a sure sign of pregnancy. As long as the line was getting stronger, it was not a 'false positive'.

"Happy Birthday, Hubberoo! Now I don't have to get you a birthday gift, right? Are you happy?" I asked him hesitantly, wondering if I could be happy if he weren't.

"Very." he said, as he gave me a big smile and kiss and then wrapped me in a tight bear hug. I was relieved and ecstatic and my heart rejoiced. I'm sure he was caught completely off guard by the whole situation just as I was, but I was apprehensive because I thought he might be unhappy. It was the perfect response from him, and I basked in the warm and fuzzy feeling that overcame me.

So, did you know that a positive result could also

be a 'false positive'? That was the first time I heard of it. What the heck is a false positive, I had wondered to myself, as I typed furiously away on the keyboard to find out on the internet search engine.

Always follow up with a doctor to make sure you're actually pregnant and to ensure you start caring for yourself and your little one properly.

- False positives don't happen too often, but they do happen. It can be caused by:
    - An 'evaporation line' – this appears when the pee in the stick starts to dry up and it leaves behind the faint tint. It can occur if you look at the stick too long after the required time. For example, if you throw it in the trash, don't go back thirty minutes later to check it again - it won't be an accurate representation of your pregnancy status. So make sure you look at the test immediately after the recommended waiting time and before the recommended time frame ends.
    - By medications that you might be on which can contaminate the urine with blood or gross amounts of protein, and may lead to inaccurate results by causing what is known as 'phantom HCG'.
- Pain Relief, Anxiety, or Meds for Nausea, Allergies, or Sleeplessness: non-fertility medications that can cause a false positive include: methadone, chlordiazepoxide, and promethazine.

- Antiepileptic or Anticonvulsants: Drugs such as barbiturates, bromides, benzodiazepines, fructose derivatives, fatty acids, triazines, primidone, GABA analogs, and other anticonvulsants can also affect the accuracy of your pregnancy test.
- Anti-Anxiety Medication and Tranquilizers: usually more common with prescription anti-anxiety medications, such as azapirones, benzodiazepines, and hydroxyzine. Psychosis management requires antipsychotics, such as chlorpromazine, droperidol, triflupromazine and clozapine, which can also affect your pregnancy test.
- Anti-Parkinson Medications: which may include tyrosine, phenylalanine, and anticholinergics such as scopolamine and benztropine.
- Diuretics: such as furosemide, thiazides, spironolactone, and osmotic diuretics, like glucose and mannitol.
  - Certain forms of cancer may elevate hCG levels and also cause false positives.
  - Defective home pregnancy tests.

3

IT IS EXTREMELY IMPORTANT TO SCHEDULE A VISIT TO SEE AN OB/GYN AS SOON AS POSSIBLE.

Our first appointment at the OB/GYN was interesting. The positive pee test was on a Friday, and the earliest doctor's appointment my husband was able to schedule was on the following Wednesday. We had gone through various websites trying to find a good OB/GYN who we thought we would feel comfortable with, and who would also be covered under my husband's health insurance plan. When we arrived at the doctor's clinic, we had to fill out a bunch of forms that asked questions about my medical history and any family history of genetic diseases such as diabetes, etc.

When we were finally face to face with our doctor, she asked a few questions and then casually asked "so what makes you think you're pregnant?"

I responded with "I took five pregnancy tests, they're all in my purse, I brought them in case you want to see them!"

She laughed and said she believed me and then made a reference to the show The Mindy Project and how the main character Mindy had a whole bunch of tests lying on her bed and was holding the one stick that had a negative result amid the remaining positives, saying "This one says I may not be pregnant after all!" It was amusing. I had never watched The Mindy Project, so we just chuckled at the scenario she described. We really wanted the baby, so the reason for my excessive number of tests was to make sure that I really was happily pregnant, and not because I was hoping we weren't. I did look up the episode when I got home and watched the scene. Then I ended up watching a whole season of the show. *Thanks, Doc.*

I had always, always had highly irregular periods, and had even gone about 5 months once without one in sight. One particularly nasty month, I had my period for an entire month straight. Yeah, I know that's not normal. I never went to the doctor to check up on it, even though everyone said I should - but I had been in enough hospitals as a young child and figured when I wanted to have kids, I'd get around to having myself examined. We weren't able to determine any possible date of conception by the last menstrual period (LMP) date because of this irregularity and it had been over a month and a half as far as I could remember since I approximately had it last. For as long as I could remember, I would get my period every other month or so. I didn't keep exact track of it. The doctor said it was most likely Polycystic Ovary Syndrome ("PCOS"). The diagnosis certainly explained why I had acne well past my teenage years! Since I didn't have regular periods, I obviously couldn't confirm the pregnancy by having a late or missed period.

"No worries, we'll just schedule an ultrasound to confirm the pregnancy and figure out the gestational age!" she said.

She scheduled an ultrasound for the next day. I didn't want to let myself be excited about it until I saw actual confirmation that I really was pregnant by seeing the little image of a fetus on the ultrasound. I didn't want to have any false hope. My husband and I eagerly counted down the hours to our appointment - we couldn't wait to see our little bean on the monitor!

4

ULTRASOUNDS CAN BE DISAPPOINTING.

The ultrasound appointment day finally arrived. I was given a little sheet full of fun facts to take home, which stated that I was to drink at least a full bottle of water the hour before our scheduled ultrasound. We sat waiting for our turn, taking selfies on our cellphones. The tech finally called us in and I was told to remove everything waist down. She also told me I could empty my bladder if I wanted to, which confused me since I thought I had to have a full bladder. Apparently, a transvaginal ultrasound works better if your bladder is empty. The standard external ultrasound device works better if your bladder is full. As an aside, I shall state that prior to my pregnancy, I had a certain degree of shyness and modesty when it came to shedding my clothing, being that I am extremely introverted and also generally hated people touching me. By the time I had given birth, I was shameless. My sister complained quite often of my immodesty and general tendency to walk around with a boob or two flailing around uncovered. It changes you, pregnancy. In more ways than one. Anyway, back to the first ultrasound - we were sorely disappointed to be told by the ultrasound tech that it was too early to see any sign of an embryo. All that was visible was the yolk sac - there was no fetal pole as yet.

5

*YOU CAN'T SEE THE EMBRYO ON AN
ULTRASOUND PRIOR TO 5 WEEKS GESTATION.*

Who knew? Just my luck. Apparently the earliest date that the fetal pole would appear on the ultrasound would be at 5 and a half weeks. We were sent home, disappointed, with another ultrasound scheduled for the following Thursday. I was freaking out a bit internally on the way home, although I didn't mention my feelings to my husband.

I had never heard of a fetal pole or a yolk sac before, and wondered what it meant for there to be one and not the other. I always thought you just saw the developing embryonic cells in an ultrasound, along with a cute umbilical cord. Nope. Of course not. I spent some time researching it and felt much better. However, I was still worried that the fetal pole might not show up the next week, and was unable to enjoy the fact that I was pregnant when all that I had confirmation of was that there was this mysterious yolk sac with nothing visible inside it. At least I knew that I was not past 6 weeks gestation at the very least, based on the fact that the fetal pole was not yet visible.

- Ultrasounds
- They use high frequency sounds waves to scan the abdomen and pelvic cavity and create a picture (sonogram) of the baby and placenta. Ultrasounds have many uses during pregnancy:
    - Determine due dates (by dating the estimated number of weeks of gestation of the fetus)
    - Reveal if there are twins or multiples
    - Rule out complications, such as ectopic pregnancies (where the embryo implants in the wrong place, such as the fallopian tubes)
    - Screen for birth defects
    - Determine position of the placenta and any related issues
    - Posterior or anterior position, whether it is too low, whether there is any placental abruption
    - Determine the position of the baby, whether it is breech or not
        - A breech baby may complicate delivery, and often results in a scheduled c-section, if an attempt by your doctor to manually turn the baby fails or is refused.
    - Determine the sex of your baby
- There are various types of ultrasounds, the basic three being:
    - Transvaginal – using an internal probe. These are most often used during the earlier stages of pregnancy and produce 2D images
    - Standard – using an external transducer to

produce 2D images
- o 3D or 4D – produces 3D or 4D images
- Yolk Sac
  - o A membrane which plays a critical role in the embryo's development
  - o It is the first structure that is seen within the gestational sac, at around 5 weeks gestation.
  - o It provides nutrition to the embryo before the placenta takes over.
  - o The yolk sac usually doesn't grow larger than 6mm – if it does, then something may be abnormal with the pregnancy.
  - o If the yolk sac is not visible when the gestational sac has grown to about 12mm, then this may indicate a failed pregnancy.
- Fetal Pole
  - o The first visible sign of a developing embryo and appears as a thickening on the margin of the yolk sac at around 5.5 weeks gestation.
  - o This is usually visible only at around 6 weeks with vaginal ultrasound imaging, and at about 8 weeks with abdominal ultrasound imaging.

6

The following Thursday finally came. Each day felt like a year to me. I was still feeling nauseous throughout the week, a queasy feeling that came and went throughout the day – it was not limited to just the mornings. I wondered when I would start throwing up like the movies always depicted. I also wondered why it wasn't called "all-day sickness", instead of "morning sickness".

This time, we were in luck. We were able to see a tiny little life growing inside of me. It looked like a little bean. The most amazing and breathtaking moment for us was when the ultrasound tech showed us a flickering motion on the ultrasound machine screen.

"That's the heartbeat," she said, pointing to the computer screen where the sound waves were depicted with bars rising and falling.

I was speechless as she let us listen to a simulated sound of the heartbeat. It was extremely fast, sounding like a supersonic train chugging along on tracks. But steady. It was the most beautiful thing I had ever heard. "How old is Little Bean?" I asked.

She responded that I was 6 weeks pregnant that day. She printed out a couple of images for us to take home. I couldn't believe that the baby's heart had already begun to beat at 6 weeks. I don't know why, but it was just amazing to have heard the sound. Life had begun, and we had created it out of what seemed like nothing. I marveled at the miracle that spark of life was. It was nothing to look at, barely resembling anything even close to a human being, and yet, it had a steadily beating heart.

7

HCG LEVELS RISE SUBSTANTIALLY DURING EARLY PREGNANCY.

"I hate you!" I yelled angrily at my husband before collapsing on the couch with a sob. "Why did you throw away the last cupcake?!"

He looked a bit stunned, "It was stale... I'll get you another one!"

"NO, I wanted THAT one!" I seethed, eyeing him with looks that shot daggers. "You're thoughtless and selfish!"

"I didn't know it was that important to you... I'll get you another one, a freshly baked one..."

"Noooo."

Too much caffeine is bad for Little Fetus, so I stopped drinking it once my pregnancy was confirmed. I was not prepared for the sudden lack of caffeine. I was apparently quite addicted to caffeine, and found myself having literal withdrawal symptoms. *This must be how drug addicts feel. I can never judge anyone again.* In other words, in addition to feeling shaky and having a headache, I was ready to kill anyone within reach. If you're planning on getting pregnant, it is probably a good idea to start weaning yourself off the coffee addiction a few months prior. The increased pregnancy hormones already made me more emotional, but combined with the lack of delicious, soothing coffee, I was, as my mother called me, a veritable 'firecracker'.

"Why does everything and everybody suck?" I questioned irritably, conjuring up visions of coffee cups around me, steaming and frothy.

Out of the corner of my eye, I could see Hubby tiptoeing backwards out of the room.

"Coffeeeeeeeeeee," I was lying spreadeagled on the couch in a mock faint, "I neeeeed coffeeeeee!" I moaned to myself and to Little Fetus.

After a few days of this, I caved in and allowed myself to have one cup of coffee a day. This was a huge drop from the usual four cups of coffee and tea I had drunk every single day for the past ten years, I consoled myself. I knew a cup a day was fine for Little Fetus, but I had really wanted to try and just cut out all caffeine cold turkey - but it was not going to happen. *For the sake of everyone around me.* It definitely dulled the irritability I felt, but I was still pretty emotional throughout my pregnancy.

"Poor Nemo," I wiped a tear from my eye. "This is so sad."

My sister just shook her head, "Oh man, is this what I'm going to be like when I'm pregnant?" she pondered out aloud. "You've watched this movie a thousand times and never cried."

"I know," I looked at her, "I can't help it. It's just making me all weepy for some reason!"

"This part of the movie isn't even sad!" she said, wide-eyed.

"But it will be later on!" I reminded her. "Foreshadowing!!"

She shook her head in wonder at what I had become.

◆◆◆

As the days went by, and the aches and pains took hold of my body, a massage seemed like it would help. I poked Hubby one night, as we lay in bed. He snorted and turned over. I poked him again.

"Huh? What?" he asked sleepily.

"WHY are you always so tired these days?!" I asked him, irritated. He had been complaining that he had body pains and was constantly tired too. I wondered if he really was having those 'sympathy symptoms' some men apparently have when their wives are pregnant. Yes, pregnancy sympathy is an actual thing - researchers have found that some fathers-to-be endure cramps, back pain, mood swings, food cravings, morning sickness, extreme tiredness, depression, irritability, fainting and toothache when their wives are pregnant. Hubby had never complained about being so tired and achy before and nothing had really changed in his routine. I was not feeling too sympathetic about his plight as I shook his arm.

"Remember that massage you offered last evening that I didn't take you up on?" I hissed.

"Yeah. You want one?" he turned back around, and started lightly massaging my neck.

"Ohh, that's perfect." I sighed happily, as he rubbed my shoulders. The rubbing got significantly lighter within a few minutes. I poked him again. He started massaging me with more pressure again.

Less than three minutes later, his fingers went limp as he fell asleep. I was livid. I pushed his hands off me angrily and threw a pillow at him. He woke up, startled and started mumbling a half-hearted apology. "I'm sorry, boo-boo... I'm just so tired. I have to go to work in the morning!"

"You've been up way later than this before and have been wide awake!" I shrieked.

"I'm sorry!" he said, "Here, let me try again!"

"NO!" I turned over and wept into my pillow. "You suck at giving massages! Don't touch me!" I mean, seriously, he had asked me for a massage three times over the last few weeks, and I had obliged. *I'd given him really good ones too*, I pouted to myself in self-pity. *And he can't give me just one proper massage?! Who's the pregnant one here?!* I vowed to never ask him for another massage again.

"That's really mean," he grumbled as he went back to sleep.

And that's when I whisked out my cell and started googling furiously on Amazon. *I don't need him for a damn massage! They have massage chairs for a reason!* As it turned out, they also have massage pillows, which are more convenient since you can just use them while you're in bed. I ordered it and waited in anticipation for it to arrive two days later.

"Ermagad" I melted into a ball of mush, "This is heavenly."

The little massage pillow was perfectly designed. It also had a heat function that spread a wonderful warmth as the internal massage balls moved around. Hubby was a little insulted, but I didn't care. "At least the people who made this pillow care about me," I huffed to my husband.

"I can't believe you said I give horrible massages" he said in response.

"Are you SERIOUSLY saying that?" I fumed, "You fell asleep five minutes in. And the other couple of times, you barely applied any pressure. So, it's true!"

"Fine!" he shot back. "Don't ask me to give you one!"

"I won't!" I yelled back, knowing in the back of my mind that we sounded like two 4 year old children but not caring.

My birthday was coming up soon and I was looking forward to seeing my parents and sister who had promised to fly in to visit. My sister and I were on FaceTime when she broke the terrible news to me.

"We won't be able to make it that weekend, the flights are too expensive. We'll come a few weeks after, okay?"

"What?!" my voice was shaking with disappointment. "Seriously?!" I had to blink back tears. I was overwhelmed with the sudden sadness I felt. *They're not coming?*

My sister's eyes widened as she immediately realized that I was upset. "Oh hey, no, I was just kidding! We're coming! We were going to surprise you and just show up!"

I could see her surprise and regret at having made me cry. "Not funny!" I managed to get out before I hung up on her.

She called back several times but I didn't answer. Later, much, much later, I found out that she had called Hubby right after, who had been driving on the way back home from work.

"Heyyy," she had said, "So, just to let you know, I did something stupid."

"Oh no." he had said.

"I was just kidding around, and wanted to surprise her and said we weren't coming. She ended up freaking out and crying." she said with an apologetic laugh, "Now she won't pick up my phone calls, so I just wanted to give you a heads up. I can't believe she's so emotional."

"Oh man." he had laugh-sighed, "You have no idea how it has been. Thanks for the heads up."

"Byeee." she had hung up, still stunned at the reaction.

My mom and sis had giggled over it for quite a while afterwards. Pregnant ladies, go figure. The pregnancy hormones make a beast out of even the most level-headed woman. I remember it took some time to get over the distress I had felt. I knew in my head that there was nothing to be upset about, but my emotions were surfacing uncontrolled. It was like I couldn't get over the initial feeling of disappointment at the thought of them not coming. My family and even my hubby had kidded around in similar fashion numerous times before and I had always found it funny and had been HAPPY when I'd figured out they were actually going to show up. Hubby had loved popping up for surprise visits while we were dating and had arranged for surprise visits from my sister on more than one occasion after I moved to the U.S. and I'd taken pretend-cancellations in stride. So, it was surprising even to myself that I found myself shedding tears uncontrollably.

A few hours later, she called again and I finally picked up. "Hey…. are you okay? I'm so sorry, I didn't mean to make you cry! I didn't think you would cry!!" my sister apologized.

"No, no, I know. Yeah." I told her sheepishly. "I don't even know why I got so upset. I just got so sad."

"I know. Remind me not to joke around with you like that again while you're preggo." she said with a smile, trying to lighten the mood.

"I know, I know." I said, rolling my eyes, "Man, I'm a mess. Just wait till you've got a bun in the oven." I had never been the weepy type so this was beyond embarrassing for me.

"Why do they call it having a bun in the oven, I've always wondered," she said.

"I can tell you exactly why." I had always wondered that myself, but the mystery was definitely solved now. "It's because your body turns into a hot oven, and it feels like your baby is the little bun baking in there. I'm so hot and sweaty all the time, I can just feel the heat emanating from me."

I didn't even know what hCG levels were before I got pregnant. I mean, I vaguely remembered learning something about it when I was in school, but for some reason the information never really stuck with me. So, here's a refresher: it stands for the hormone human chorionic gonadotropin, and is produced during pregnancy. The pregnancy test measures the amount of this hormone that is present in your pee.

This hGC is responsible for elevating your estrogen and progesterone hormones, which is part of the cause of magnified emotions and mood swings during pregnancy.

- hCG is produced during pregnancy by cells that form in the placenta (the placenta nourishes the egg after the egg has been fertilized and has subsequently attached to the uterine wall).
- The hormone is produced by the placenta as soon as implantation happens (about one week after fertilization)
- hCG levels approximately double about every 2 days until about 10 – 12 weeks gestation, after which they level off.
- hCG is responsible for keeping estrogen and progesterone pregnancy hormones at their appropriate levels until the placenta has developed enough to take over this function.
  - The increased levels of these pregnancy hormones are partly responsible for the

magnification of your emotions and your noticeable mood swings

- hCG increases blood supply to your pelvis, which makes your bladder want to get rid of the tiniest amount of pee.
- hCG is responsible for your morning sickness (which usually peaks at around the 8th to 10th week of pregnancy)

True enough, around my 9th week of pregnancy, I was finally throwing up in the mornings, instead of just being nauseous all day. This lasted only a week or so.

At one point I was waking up at night to rush to the washroom and throw up. I remember one especially horrible throwing up session, Hubby came in to make sure I was okay. He gently pulled back my hair out of my face so that it wouldn't get dirty. I appreciated the gesture although I shooed him out fairly quickly – I didn't like the thought of being seen throwing up. I wondered how he didn't throw up just watching me.

"Out! Out, I don't like you seeing me throw up." I gasped in between hurling. I had to practically shove him back out the door, "I'm fine, really."

"Okay, let me know if you need me." he said as he left.

"It's totally normal," my dad had assured us. "It's a great sign, actually, it means your pregnancy is progressing as it should! I'm going to make you a ginger tea, and maybe you'll feel better."

Ugh. I hate vomiting.

8

My mom's first child was stillborn. This is not the same as a miscarriage, but it certainly had a lot to do with the amount of stress I experienced due to fearing that something would go wrong with my own pregnancy. I felt like I was being quite the pessimist because none of the other moms-to-be ever expressed miscarriage as being a huge fear of theirs. It seemed to me that every other mom-to-be was just extremely joyful and happy about their pregnancy the moment they found out that they were pregnant. Or else, they were already confidently thinking of baby names and planning out all the details of how baby would be brought home and what would happen immediately after the birth. I wasn't. I couldn't bring myself to think that far.

I was constantly worrying that something I did or didn't do would possibly cause a miscarriage. Or worse, that it would cause a stillborn baby. I wasn't able to be a hundred percent happy and I knew I wouldn't be until I was holding my baby in my hands. It didn't help that I read up on the subject and managed to dig up countless numbers of stories of things going wrong. I made the same mistake in the past when I was contemplating laser eye surgery to correct my vision, which isn't terrible, but I have a pair of glasses I occasionally need to wear, which is annoying. I searched on YouTube for laser eye correction videos and saw the most horrifying ones, of course. Silly me. I still refuse to get it until the procedure doesn't require that a flap be cut out of your eyeball. But, I digress. Miscarriages... I was extra careful, as a result, to make sure that I didn't put myself in risky situations and to make sure that the food I ate was safe.

My husband and I were supposed to go go-karting the weekend we found out I was pregnant. It was part of Hubby's birthday celebrations. Needless to say, I didn't end up going. I wasn't entirely sure if it was a good idea to even go, so I did a little research on the subject:

- Placental Abruption: is when the placenta breaks away (abrupts) from the wall of the uterus too early. This can be very harmful. In rare cases, it can be deadly. The baby could be born prematurely or the mother could lose a lot of blood. Trauma to your abdomen — such as from a fall, car accident, or any type of situation resulting in a blow to the abdomen — makes placental abruption more likely. It is harder to diagnose placental abruption before the 20th week of pregnancy because the placenta is so small. Separation can be a temporary problem or it can lead to a miscarriage.

[41]

- However, many sources cited that a baby in the womb is actually very well protected. In the first trimester, a thick, muscular uterus and an even more protective pelvic bone shield your baby, so it is nearly impossible to injure Little Fetus if you trip and fall. It takes a really hard fall to injure the baby - the kind which injures the mom.

So, apparently, the Little Fetus is very well protected and many women have chosen to go skiing, go-karting, marathon running, or on amusement park rides during their pregnancies. Nevertheless, I, on the other hand, chose to stay home and undertake my own version of a marathon – a Netflix marathon watching session.

Life, of course, has its ways of throwing you for a loop, regardless of all the caution and precautions you take. Knowing this information didn't make it any easier on me when our dog, which had now grown into an 80 lb furball, jumped on me in excitement one day after I returned from The Upstairs, after being away for a grand total of 5 minutes (aka. "Forever" in dog terms). She pawed me right in the belly when I sat on the couch, right where Little Fetus was. I was horrified and started googling frantically on the subject. 'All will be well, Mama,' was the general theme of the results. I was unsettled for a long while afterwards, wondering if there could be any sort of damage to Little Fetus. Moms on online forums had many similar stories to share, except the stories were mostly recounting incidents of their toddlers jumping on their pregnant bellies or accidentally kicking them. For the record, Little Fetus turned out to be just fine.

It's perplexing, the types of things that can happen to you when you're pregnant, or perhaps it is just the way of the world – the more you try to be careful, the more dangerous things you get yourself into. I found myself to be a little clumsier and more forgetful than usual, perhaps just from being more tired throughout the day. One morning, as I was cleaning the kitchen, I decided to boil some water in a "One Shot" kettle - it boils just enough water for one cup as fast as ever. It's the best little kettle, since nothing annoys me more than having to wait forever for water to boil. In the meantime, I was wiping the kitchen counters and somehow forgot that I had just filled it to the brim and turned it on. I picked it up with one hand and was unable to balance it so it fell over and all that boiling water spilled onto my arm. I shrieked in surprise more than in pain.

I immediately stuck my hand under some cold water and held it there for a while. Hubby had jumped up to come see what happened and was frantically looking around for some ointment to put on my arm. We couldn't find any. *Note to self, stock up on first aid supplies.*

"Try ice!" Hubby suggested.

"Nope, ice is supposed to make it worse, isn't it?" I said, "Cold water will prevent blisters."

"What happened?!"

"I don't know. I was just clumsy," I sighed. My arm felt like it was burning from the inside.

The cold water wasn't helping much. I suddenly remembered that aloe vera is supposed to be extremely soothing and healing for burns, and luckily for me, we had a giant aloe vera plant in the house that managed to stay alive.

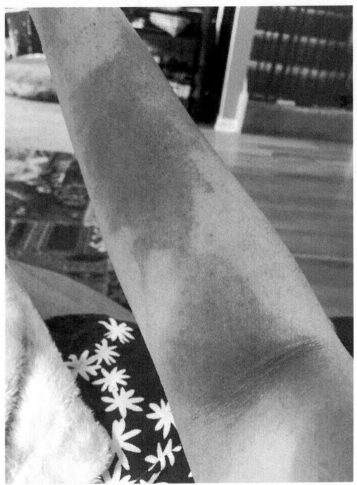

"Aloe vera!" I exclaimed!

Hubby didn't look too convinced, but went to get the plant.

"I don't know if I'm doing this right," Hubby said nervously as he cut one of the leaves and exposed the soft, wet gel-like inner pulp of the plant. He rubbed this gel on my arm. It had an immediate cooling feel and my arm no longer felt like it was on fire.

A week later, my arm looked like I had bruised it badly, but it only looked terrible - I felt no pain at all and continued to apply a little bit of aloe vera on it. The burn discoloration took a few more months to fade away.

My husband and I had told our siblings about my pregnancy right away. However, we had waited until our ultrasound appointment confirmed the pregnancy at 6 weeks to tell our parents, and then waited the standard 12 weeks to tell everyone else that we were expecting our first child.

Are you wondering how we told my parents? No? I'm going to tell you anyway. We drove to their home (an 8 hour drive) without telling them and walked into the house. We brought our dog with us, and it set off the two dogs they had. There was maddening barking for a while as my parents' dogs had never met our dog before and were being territorial. We probably should have rung the doorbell instead of just walking in through the unlocked door, come to think of it. My parents were caught so off guard that they just walked slowly to the front entrance and looked at Hubby and I without speaking. I don't think they recognized us for a minute.

"Hi! Surprise!" I hugged them both.

"What are you doing here?" my dad asked, scratching his head. He had an allergic reaction to some hair dye he had used, which was why he was scratching.

"We brought you a cake!" Hubby responded.

"Why weren't you guys more concerned about the dogs barking like that?" I inquired, shaking my head in disapproval. "If we had been burglars, you'd have been in trouble."

"Bah." My mom replied as she peered into the box that held the cake. She took it out and put it on the kitchen island. They squinted, trying to read the words written in icing on the cake.

"What does that say?" They asked, "Congrats, garage what?"

I rolled my eyes and sighed dramatically. This wasn't going the way I had planned.

"It says, 'Congrats, Grandma and Grandpa!'"

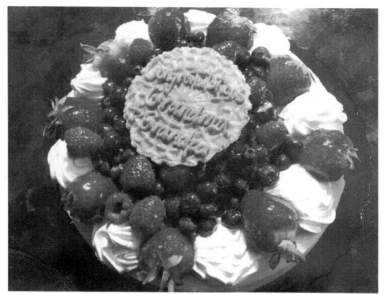

"Oh," they looked confused for a minute. I was in disbelief. They're normally quite quick and have sharp minds.

I attributed it to the fact they had just been awoken from their evening nap and were also still trying to process the fact that we had arrived out of the blue from Chicago and ended on their doorstep in Toronto without warning.

"Ohhhhhhh!" it finally sunk in, and their faces brightened and smiles widened. The cake was delicious. My parents were deliriously happy, as it would be their first grandchild. I cried happy tears of joy.

About halfway through my pregnancy, I posted an announcement on Facebook, it was just a photo taken randomly – no professional photo shoot - with the caption "Halfway there!". I was not entirely surprised when some older relatives had apparently commented to my mother that I shouldn't have announced my pregnancy to everyone.

What if she has a problem with the pregnancy? With the baby?

I dismissed their concerns. I already was paranoid about things going wrong, but at this point if something went wrong, would people expect me to pretend as if I had never been pregnant at all? To dismiss the fact that a beautiful little baby with a beating heart and growing body and brain existed within me? Her life had already begun, as far as I was concerned.

In the midst of all of this, we decided to move from our two-bedroom condo without a backyard to a four-bedroom house in the suburbs with a backyard for Doggy. We had quite a bit of stress during this transition, especially with figuring out mortgage options and deciding whether or not we could keep the condo as an investment property. It added a lot of stress to my pregnancy experience.

It also didn't help when, less than a week before we were finally moving to the new house, we decided to take Doggy out for a walk around the neighborhood and she ended up biting another dog's ear off, Mike Tyson style.

Yep, she bit that dog's ear off.

It was a giant, fat, energetic golden Labrador. Its owner had absolutely no control over it, and we saw it dragging its owner from a mile away. Knowing that our Doggy was quite reactive, especially due to my pregnancy, Hubby and I moved to the very edge of the sidewalk and parked her furry butt on the grass.

"She's in training," we stated pleasantly as DroolyLab dragged its owner towards us.

"Oh, he's friendly!" she chirped at us, tugging unsuccessfully at his leash in an attempt to restrain him.

"She's not friendly," I warned, "Don't let your dog come any closer."

"Oh, okay," she panted, still tugging unsuccesfully at his leash, "but don't worry, he just wants to say hi."

Hubby moved to stand in front of both me and Doggy. Our dog was still sitting calmly, a good distance away from the sidewalk to allow them to pass without the dogs being within physical contact. Although she was calm and stationary, she had her eyes glued to the DroolyLab, watching him like a hawk. Hubby was holding on to her leash. Hubby was unable to stop DroolyLab from bounding towards our dear Doggy and lunging at her face. Doggy reacted instantly and nipped at DroolyLab, who yelped in surprise and jumped back.

It was only then that DroolyLab's owner was able to pull him away, heaving and huffing. Hubby pulled Doggy's leash back as she started barking at DroolyLab. The owner was still smiling as she said "Oh, so sorry! He's okay! Have a great day!" and made her way to her condo which was just in front of us.

"That won't be the last we see of them," I murmured to Hubby.

"Ah, it looked fine." he replied.

"Mark my words," I said, "they're going to come ask us for money."

Sure enough, that night, the owner's husband knocked on our door and asked us to pay for half of their dog's vet bill, which came up to about $600. Apparently, our dog had ripped off a tiny piece of DroolyLab's ear, which required surgery. We hadn't noticed any blood at the scene, but they provided vet bills for us to look at, so we paid it, but it was additional stress we just didn't need.

"We couldn't find his ear piece that was torn off. I looked around." The owner's husband said, as he handed us the vet bill.

The timing couldn't have been worse, as we were closing on our house that week - a week later, and our cute Doggy would've never have even met DroolyLab. She had never bitten any other dog before, so it was unfortunate, to say the least. But I knew that she had been provoked into it, as she had been calm and stationary right up until DroolyLab's owner had allowed her dog (which must have looked like a giant stampeding beast in our Doggy's eyes) to physically jump onto ours and in such close proximity to my pregnant self.

9

YOU CAN HEAR YOUR BABY'S HEARTBEAT IN THE PRIVACY OF YOUR OWN HOME.

The fetal doppler brought the greatest sense of peace to my mind. Everyone I asked before I purchased it recommended that I not buy it. It is a small portable device that allows you to hear your baby's heartbeat for yourself, in the privacy of your own home, rather than having to wait till you see a doctor. You can purchase one easily almost anywhere these days.

Most of the concerns (even by people on the internet forums) against buying one were because people believed that if the mother-to-be bought one and for some reason couldn't find or hear the fetal heartbeat, she'd be more stressed. Apparently, a lot of times the baby would move to a position that made it harder to hear its heartbeat, or else the baby's general position could make it hard to hear it at all. I decided to chance it anyway.

I purchased the Sonaline B Fetal Doppler when I was in my 11th week, and it was great - I was able to find the heartbeat each time. I would put it to my heart first just so I would know the difference, then searched around for Little Fetus' heartbeat. It was much faster than mine, and sounded like a steam engine chugging along. Some days it would take me less than a minute to find it, other days it would take perhaps 15 minutes or more. If you don't hear it occasionally, it is best to just wait for an hour and then try again. I figured if I didn't hear the heartbeat for more than half a day, I would head to the doctor's office. Thankfully, after a few hours I would hear it again.

I tried not to listen for the heartbeat more than once or twice a day, just in case it were to affect the baby in some way. It isn't dangerous to the baby, but I figured it was probably best to try and limit the baby's exposure to the ultrasound waves.

- The fetal heart Doppler works by emitting and receiving continuous ultrasound waves and then emitting the shift in frequency and wavelength.
- For some women, the fetal heart can be detected as early as 8-12 weeks.
- Most Dopplers can't reliably detect a baby's heartbeat until 10 to 12 weeks

10

YOU WILL NOT KNOW THAT YOU ARE HAVING MOOD SWINGS AND CRAVINGS.

Your significant other will tread cautiously around you, and only once you have given birth to the baby will they admit to you that they were relieved that all your mood swings and general emotional upheavals were attributed to your pregnancy. If they are smart, they will not have mentioned this at all during your pregnancy. If they are really smart, they will make you smiley face dinners to boost your mood.

My hubby was awesome at making me smile. Here's a picture of a mashed potato, steak and asparagus dinner he presented me with one night.

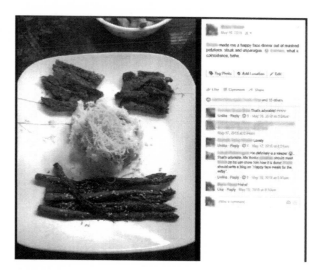

My parents and sister were also really careful about what they said around me. My brother was living abroad so he was spared the emotions of the preggo sister. My parents were afraid they would set me off unexpectedly into a weeping sobbing pile of tears so they kept conversation to a minimum. My mom spoiled me rotten. She cooked all my favourite food and brought it to my bedside or the couch. I'd get a delicious milky coffee every morning made the way only she could make it. My dad would cook my favourite chicken and potato curry and yell at me to hold on to the staircase railings every time I waddled down the stairs, holding my belly instead.

I think the most adorable thing that happened was that my dad came home one day to find me sitting on his favourite leather recliner - his throne. He scratched his itchy head, looking at me with a big smile on his face, then sat down on one of the other couches. I offered his throne back, but he refused. I don't know why, but I found it to be a really endearing memory. My sister was my personal chauffeur and assistant and all-around comforter. We'd stay up late at night and watch Netflix many a night.

One of the best things my mom forced me to do was to buy maternity clothes and maternity undies. I protested quite a bit before giving in — my mother was insistent and practically dragged me into a maternity store. The first thing the lady at the store said was "You need to be sized for a bigger bra." She took my measurements and provided me with the right sized underwear. It was such a good fit, I was finally able to breathe normally.

"I thought my breathing problem was just a pregnancy side-effect." I said.

She laughed me, and said, "Oh, aren't you a dear. You've got a wonderful mom for her to drag you in here."

"I do." I admitted. "I can't believe how comfortable I feel." I practically skipped out of the store with joy.

"So, do you have any cravings yet?" a friend asked me one day.

"Nope! Oddly enough, I don't." I stated matter-of-factly.

"Uh, YES, she does." My sister interrupted our conversation. I looked at her in surprise.

"I do?" I asked, furrowing my brows trying to remember when I had and coming up blank.

"You asked me to make you a sandwich a few nights ago at 1 am with breaded chicken cutlets, mayo and hot sauce."

"And you've been craving fast food burgers and fries non-stop, before this you hardly ate fast food anymore!" my husband chimed in, "She asked for some Mc D fries at 10 pm one night!"

"Oh yeaaaah," I said, surprised that I hadn't connected these as being cravings, or that I hadn't realized that they had been out of the norm for me. "I blame it on PreggoBrain."

"Preggowhat?" my friend asked with a laugh.

"PreggoBrain," I repeated. "My brain has been turned to mush. I can't remember anything and my thoughts are kinda sluggish. The other day I put the remote control in the fridge and another time I put my cell phone in the microwave instead of my cup!"

"And she also walked around for 20 minutes one day asking me where her reading glasses were." My sister chuckled, "I had to point out that she was wearing them."

"I've never seen her eat so much cereal," my mom joined in the conversation.

"Every night," My sister agreed, "and she always

[58]

gets hungry around 11pm. I'll hear her rummaging through the fridge right on cue."

"I didn't even realize I was doing any of that," I laughed. "Food just makes me happy. Well, happier than it normally does."

11

YOUR BODY WILL CHANGE, AND IT WILL EXPEND ENORMOUS AMOUNTS OF ENERGY TRYING TO GROW A BABY.

The first major thing I noticed was how incredibly exhausted I was. It wasn't until I started taking the prenatal vitamins that I was able to actually function. I always thought that the prenatal vitamins were solely for the health of the baby, but to a large extent they also fuel your own body. Prenatal vitamins also cause unpleasant side-effects, if you're unlucky. I noticed I was a lot more nauseous after I took them. I didn't bother to change to a different brand, and so I can't tell you if that would have helped.

At one point, I fell asleep in the car. Now, I have to admit, when I fall asleep, my mouth tends to hang open. So, there I was, sitting in the driver's seat of the car, parked in the parking lot, waiting for my mom to come back from Home Depot, where I'd driven her to for a quick shopping trip to pick up some weed killer spray. I was exhausted and it wasn't too long before I fell asleep at the wheel. I can only imagine what I must have looked like while I dozed off, mouth gaping wide open, slumped backwards in my seat, eyes closed and radio on. A hard tap at the window woke me up and I jerked awake, startled.

A middle aged man was standing there, and he jumped as he realized I was not actually dead or unconscious as he obviously must have thought. He said, "Oh! You're okay!" and walked quickly away without giving me time to respond.

I was quite embarassed. But definitely not dead. *What a nice man, I can't believe he actually came to check.* I'd probably have just walked on by.

12

CONSUMING A LITTLE ALCOHOL DURING THE FIRST FEW WEEKS IS NOT GUARANTEED TO HARM YOUR BABY.

During the first 4 weeks that I didn't know I was pregnant, I had indulged in a shot of Hennessy, or a mix of Sprite and Vodka or a glass of red wine for several nights during the weeks. I was sick to my stomach worrying about possible birth defects due to this. I brought it up with my OB/GYN and she assured me that it would be fine as long as I had only had a minimal amount to drink during each week. I had never had enough to drink to the point that I had ever been drunk, so the baby should be fine, she said. She said that the modern books and advice we seem to be getting these days concerning a zero alcohol policy during pregnancy are a bit extreme and a glass of wine here and there would be fine. There are several studies undertaken by researchers that give conflicting information regarding this, so I was still uneasy. However, Little Fetus turned out to be just fine and has an excellent memory and no physical or mental abnormalities.

I was paranoid for almost a year after she was born, truth be told, and was not able to rest easy until she started hitting all her milestones without any problems. A little blurb that made me feel a little better after countless hours of research concerned where exactly the developing embryo gets its nutrients from during the first 3-4 weeks of pregnancy: it gets it from the yolk sac. Then, once the placenta is fully formed the placenta will take over the transfer of nutrients to the embryo. So, once the placenta is formed, if you continue drinking, the baby will then be ingesting the alcohol as well. The alcohol will have the worst effect once the yolk sac is gone. I am not too sure of the accuracy of this, although it was cited in a somewhat reputable looking medical site. In other words, don't rely on the preceding information, and take it with a handful of grains of salt.

I immediately stopped drinking the moment I found out I was pregnant. Risks associated with drinking during pregnancy:

- Heavy use of alcohol during pregnancy has been linked to a long-term and irreversible condition known as fetal alcohol syndrome (FAS).
    - Babies with FAS may be born early, are often underweight and don't grow well. Some have characteristic facial features like a thin upper lip and small eye openings, or the small vertical groove between the upper lip and the nose may be flattened.

Other physical signs include a small head, short nose, and problems with the way the heart or the joints are formed.

o Children with FAS are slower to learn language skills than other kids. Often, learning disabilities and difficulty with attention, memory and hyperactivity are evident when they reach school age. They are more likely to have poor coordination and poor problem-solving skills. Some have trouble socially and find it difficult to make friends and relate to other kids.

- A study done on mice by researchers apparently demonstrated that early exposure to alcohol created changes in the expression of genes in the brains of the infant mice. These changes were observed in the hippocampus, a brain region associated with learning, memory and emotion that is known to be heavily affected by alcohol. The researchers also found changes in the bone marrow of the infant mice, and in some tissue within the mouse's snout that plays a role in the sense of smell. The researchers explained that early pregnancy is a critical time for cell division and differentiation and the embryo is vulnerable to external influences at this stage, and therefore any changes can become widespread because the cells are rapidly dividing. This demonstrated that the effects of alcohol on the embryo "cause life-long changes in brain structure, function, and behavior." However, it has not been determined just how much alcohol consumption is considered to be safe or unsafe - other than to specify that excessive drinking is definitely unsafe.

- Excessive alcohol consumption may lead to miscarriage or stillbirth, according to some sources.

Because brain growth takes place throughout pregnancy, the sooner you stop drinking the safer it will be for you and your baby.

The most odd part of my pregnancy was that I craved alcohol more than usual. This was odd mainly because I was never the type of person to drink much – I was mostly a social drinker. Even the amount that I had been drinking during these first four weeks was out of the norm for me – I had been craving a drink of wine more than usual. Once I found out I was pregnant, that craving magnified ten-fold. I wondered if the mere prohibition on drinking alcohol was responsible for the unusual craving. Some nights, as my hubby would have a drink with his dinner, I'd stare at his glass. It would be calling my name, and whispering, *drink me.* Okay, not literally, but you get what I mean, right?

13

A tipped uterus is actually a thing. And the back pain you expect to have at the end of your third trimester can actually be an issue during your first trimester. One in five women have a "tipped", "tilted" or "retroverted" uterus.

Guess who had one? Yes. I did.

It resulted in really horrible back pain starting during week 7 and lasting up until week 12. It was so bad that I had trouble walking and trouble standing for long periods of time. I didn't know you could get back pain so early on during pregnancy when the Little Fetus is nothing more than a tiny speck in your womb. Neither did a lot of other people - I got the raised eyebrow and surprised "Really!" when I mentioned the horrible back pain being the reason why I was unable to enjoy my usual activities. Most people, including myself, hadn't heard of a tipped uterus unless they were in the medical field. My OB/GYN was able to tell just by a physical exam.

When I did research it, many women were also fortunate enough to not be affected at all by the tipped uterus. In my case, it seemed that it was tipping more into my spine than most. The good news, as I was informed by my OB/GYN, was that by weeks 12-14, it would automatically right itself and it would no longer be an issue. Right on cue, by week 12 I was able to resume all my normal activities instead of curling up into a little ball on the bed or couch trying to relieve the pain.

I normally hate taking painkillers and I was more afraid than ever to take any for fear of harming Little Fetus, so I didn't pop any pills. A lifesaver was this wondrous invention called the "Snoogle" that my sister bought for me the moment she realized I was having depressive moments and sleepless nights due to the back pain. She had seen in on a YouTube vlogger channel that she followed and thought it might help me.

I can't even begin to tell you how much comfort and relief this one pregnancy pillow gave me. It just fit my body perfectly and I was in sleep-heaven. My sister took a picture moments after handing the pillow to me — I'd begun snoring almost immediately and slept soundly for a good number hours for the first time in a while.

I still use the Snoogle occasionally even now - more than a year postpartum.

Some symptoms if you have a tipped uterus:

- more back pain during the first trimester
- difficulty emptying bladder
  - Some doctors say that in very rare cases, if your growing uterus is tilted very far backwards during pregnancy it could push against your bladder, making it difficult to empty. You may find relief by leaning backwards when you're peeing, which may relieve any pressure by shifting your uterus off your bladder.
- a harder time locating your baby
  - There's a small chance your doctor may have trouble finding your baby with a transabdominal ultrasound, simply because your Little Fetus is a bit farther away.
  - Your doctor may use a transvaginal ultrasound to get a better look.

As your baby grows in the first trimester, your uterus expands in the pelvic cavity and by weeks 12 - 14, it will pop up out of your pelvis and into your abdomen in order to accommodate your growing baby. At this point, a retroverted uterus nearly always rights itself upwards.

Second Trimester

YOUR BABY IS EVESDROPPING

The second trimester of your pregnancy begins week 13 and goes all the way through week 27. At about week 18, your baby starts to hear sounds! It is really quite amazing to know that your baby can not only hear you, but will most likely remember many of the sounds it heard in the womb after birth.

After birth, at less than one week of age, my baby would immediately stop crying when I played a certain favourite song of mine that I had often played while pregnant. We first discovered this while we were on our way to the pediatrician in the car. She hated that carseat, and made it known loud and clear. After about almost ten minutes of non-stop crying, and having tried everything we could from shaking rattles to singing songs and making silly faces, we finally put the music on the radio. Soothing classical music. Jazz. Easy listening. How about the top hits station?

Nope. She was still crying.

Then I decided to soothe my own nerves by streaming music from my cell via bluetooth. The first song that came on was my most played favourite song - the one I would play constantly when she was in my womb. She stopped crying immediately. We were astonished, and relieved. And happy. She fell asleep within minutes, lulled by the fast latin pop beat. Yeah, it didn't make any sense to me either. *Forget soothing lullabies and soft music, mom.*

Little Fetus was also exposed to frequent vacuum cleaner sounds, loud voices, music and movies, and dog barking. When she was born, I believe all the chaos she heard while in the womb had desensitized her to the point that she was a relatively 'chill' baby.

By about week 25, your baby will begin to respond to sounds that are heard - kicking and moving in response to external stimuli.

15

*YOUR LITTLE ONE WILL KICK AND PUNCH
YOU GLEEFULLY AND YOU MAY BE ABLE TO SEE
THEIR LIMBS PUSHING YOUR BELLY OUTWARDS.*

There's nothing quite as awe inspiring as the first time you feel your baby move inside of you. Don't be surprised if you have to wonder if it is just a tummy rumble or gas. After it happens for a few weeks, you will be able to easily recognize it.

It is life-changing. It makes you really feel the miracle that is life - a tiny bunch of cells have come together to create a tiny human that will eventually breath, run, talk, play, and throw things at your head. And it is making its first movements inside of you, warmed, nourished and grown by your body.

This awe doesn't last for too long though - by the time you're ready to give birth, you'll have spent many a sleepless night being poked in the rib by a random fetal hand or leg, unable to breathe when they have grown to the size of a whale inside of you and kicking and punching with a vigor best described as superman on steroids having a battle inside of you with a pretend foe. So, enjoy that feeling while it lasts - savor that light, beautiful flutter of a movement and bask in the glory of you.

I remember the exact moment I was finally 100% sure that it was Little Fetus moving and not just gas that I was feeling. Hubby and I were cruising down the highway, listening to music and just chatting with each other. We were in the middle lane of a three-lane highway. On the left were three more lanes of traffic moving in the opposite direction. A medium height concrete highway dividing wall separated the two flows of traffic. All of a sudden, my husband started slowing the car down. I looked up at him and then followed his gaze.

To my absolute horror, a deer had run across the three lanes of fast moving traffic on the opposite side of the highway. By the time I looked toward it, the deer had scaled the divider and was trying to make it's way across our lanes of traffic to get to the other side. Cars started swerving all around us and I let out a gasp as the SUV in front of us, which I could see had two young children in the backseat, slammed into the concrete divider and bounced in the air before landing back on the road and sliding to a stop. The deer was right in front of us now, in the middle lane, and Hubby tapped the brakes harder, tilting the steering wheel in an attempt to avoid hitting the deer while glancing at the rearview mirror to make sure we weren't going to be hit by another car from behind.

We hit the deer.

Luckily, Hubby had reacted in time and we were traveling at a slow enough speed that the impact was minimal. However, it was still a hard enough hit that the car jolted and the poor deer staggered onto the last lane. I was petrified that an airbag would deploy and slam against my stomach. My heart was thumping in my chest so hard and I had a tingling sensation all through my body. Little Fetus immediately responded by moving the most she ever had inside of me. That flurry type feeling I wondered about possibly being gas instead of Little Fetus was most definitely the baby. I felt her move the moment we hit the deer and I had felt like my heart had jumped all the way up to my mouth. I felt like someone was tickling me with their knuckles from the inside of my lower belly. Probably not the greatest description of the little one's startled movement, but I don't know how else to describe it. My sudden rush of adrenaline and quick yell of "Eeek!" most likely prompted it. It was a scary episode.

We came to a stop on the far left shoulder, about 30 feet behind the SUV that had hit the divider wall. A few other vehicles had stopped here and there too.

"Are you okay?" Hubby grabbed my shoulders and squeezed my arms. "I'm so sorry! I couldn't avoid hitting it. Are you hurt?!" he looked panicked, even though his voice was fairly calm in tone.

"What happened to the deer?!" I peered

backwards over my shoulder, my mouth gaping as I heard more squealing tires.

"Who cares about the deer! Are you okay?!" he prodded again.

"I'm fine... No, it's okay. You did amazing. I didn't even notice that deer till it was almost in front of us. We are so lucky you saw it when you did. Oh my gawd, I felt her move like crazy!" I then suddenly exclaimed, "there were kids in that SUV! We should check them."

"You're right," he said as he hopped out of our car. I pulled myself out of our car as well and we made our way over to the SUV ahead to make sure that the family was fine. They were, thankfully and we headed back to our car. The car hood and bumper on passenger side were badly damaged and the headlight was hanging off. I looked towards the area the deer had been heading and noted sadly that it had been hit again by another car and was lying either dead or dying on the road. Some people had gotten out of their cars and were trying to move it to the far right shoulder. *Poor little deer, I thought to myself. He made it all the way across 5 lanes of traffic and we were the ones to hit it first.* I felt a sense of guilt and sadness over the loss of the deer's life.

This was the first time in my life I had ever been party to the death of an animal while in a vehicle. No, wait. I just remembered. My dad accidentally ran over a squirrel once while he was driving. That was a sad day too. I was about 15 years old at the time, in the backseat. I didn't remember that at the time of this deer incident, though. I rubbed my pregnant belly and silently thanked the heavens or whatever above that things had not been as bad for us. Hubby and I continued on our way, much more cautiously.

I think the most creepy moment in baby movement happened to me one night as I lay in bed by myself. I rolled over onto my tummy and after a few moments I clearly felt movement. It felt as if Little Fetus was turning around completely inside of me, crawling inside of me, fingers facing my belly button and palming against the inside of my belly. Perhaps she didn't like the position I had moved to. I hastily turned onto my back again.

I have to admit, in the middle of the night, in the dark, and all alone at that moment, I was more than a little creeped out - it felt like there was an alien or something inside of me and I instantly regretted having watched the movies Alien and Spaceballs when I was younger.

As I moved into the final weeks of my pregnancy during the third trimester, Little Fetus would respond quite vigorously to my gentle pokes and calls of "Hellooo, baby? Wake up!". My entire belly could be seen moving by what could only have been little baby feet and hands flailing about in response. My mother was not at all pleased by this behaviour of mine and demanded that I "stop poking that child!" She was worried I might poke its eye or something... so I eventually stopped nudging my belly.

16

"Did you know you have a giant skin tag on your neck?" I asked my sister.

"Uh, yeah." she replied.

"I could just yank it off you," I offered. "Just pull it right off for you."

"You leave Alfred alone, you weirdo," she said, "Pregnancy has really made you weirder than usual."

"I'm just saying, you can rip it off and it will be gone forever."

"Yeah, I think I'll just get that taken care by a medical professional."

"Hrmph." I mock-sulked.

You may get skin tags as a result of your pregnancy. I was never informed of this and was quite dismayed to see them popping up around my chest area. It is the result of all those hormones inside of you. They kept getting larger, and I eventually started just pulling them right off. It didn't bleed or anything, but I don't recommend you do the same. Just in case. If they really bother you, you can have them removed by a professional.

I didn't feel any pain when I ripped mine off - grabbed them by my fingernails and quickly yanked them off. It was strangely satisfying, like watching blackheads being pulled off from a Biore nose strip - you really shouldn't, but you do anyway.

There were at least 20 that popped up. They started out like tiny specks and gradually kept growing until I plucked them off. What I had always thought was a birthmark on my chest suddenly developed into a skin tag. It became raised off my skin and then started getting larger, until it looked like an odd sort of flat mushroom. I picked it off last, and that one did hurt and bleed a little. There isn't a birthmark there anymore. It must've been a really flat mole.

17

YOUR ARMPITS CAN START DARKENING NOTICEABLY, AND YOUR SKIN COLOUR IN GENERAL MAY DARKEN A FEW SHADES.

"**W**hat happened to your armpit?" my mom asked curiously.

I was wearing a sleeveless top and I had lifted my arm to comb my hair.

She saw my darkened skin. "Do you have a rash?"

"No, it's a pregnancy side effect, apparently."

"I never had that happen to me," she responded.

"Yeah? Hmm," I had to look it up, "I guess maybe its because your natural skin tone is a lot lighter than mine. I probably have more melanin production."

Another surprise. During pregnancy, thanks to an

increased production of estrogen, your body begins to produce extra melanin, which is a skin darkening pigment. This causes certain areas of your body to get darker during pregnancy. It does not hurt and is not harmful. It is really ugly to look at though.

I found myself feeling a bit self-conscious wearing sleeveless blouses and dresses. I kept moisturizing it daily, but that didn't help much. There's really nothing you can do about this during your pregnancy - you'll just have to wait till after you give birth for the skin to go back to its regular color. My entire body turned a couple of shades darker, as if I had a light tan, come to think of it.

18

YOUR NAVEL LINE WILL ALSO START DARKENING
AS YOUR PREGNANCY PROGRESSES.

This was probably one of the first visual cues I had of my pregnancy. A dark line, termed the linea nigra, was visible all the way down my stomach, starting from my navel and extending downward. As my pregnancy progressed, the line became a little more visible traveling upward from my navel almost to my ribs. This is also due to a hormonal response and increase in melanin. It lightened a couple of months after Little Fetus was born and went back to normal eventually.

19

YOU CAN GET A TEMPORARY FORM OF DIABETES - GESTATIONAL DIABETES. IT GOES AWAY ONCE THE PREGNANCY IS DONE.

If you're unlucky, you'll get Gestational Diabetes. And then you can't justify eating all the chocolate and ice cream you want anymore. If you've got some luck left over regardless, you can diet-control your gestational diabetes by simply eating in a very controlled manner. It is a complete lifestyle change if you are not used to eating healthily and exercising consistently.

Yes, I was one of the unlucky ones. Very unlucky, as I was unable to diet-control it.

For me, it was a drastic change. I was completely blindsided by the diagnosis, not even knowing that it was something that ever happened. Why had nobody ever told me this was a possibility? My father had diabetes, and I always assumed I would get it eventually some day since I was probably genetically predisposed to get it, but I never thought there was also a "temporary" type of diabetes related to pregnancy. I always had the movie version of being pregnant in my head - being able to eat and drink anything I craved as a matter of pregnancy privilege!

20

YOU MAY HAVE TO TAKE INSULIN TO CONTROL THE GESTATIONAL DIABETES IF YOUR BLOOD SUGAR LEVELS REMAIN HIGH DESPITE A CONTROLLED DIET.

I had to go to the hospital so much more after this; I felt like that's all I was doing. Once diagnosed with gestational diabetes, for each week up until Little Fetus was out of me, I had to go once a week to each of the dietician, the endocrinologist, and the ob/gyn's office. I had a minimum of 3 appointments a week. Combined with the anatomy scans, to make sure that the Little Fetus was developing normally, it seemed like I was always heading to the hospital/doctor's office. This was a little overwhelming for someone who generally hated the memories of being in hospitals as a child – when I was younger, I had a terrible immune system and would frequently be taken to the doctor by my parents due to various ailments.

I had decided to stay at my parent's home for the last 3 months of my pregnancy so that I could be spoiled by my mom and sister, so I was lucky that I had them available to drive me to all these appointments and to support me in general. Eventually, I was unable to control my diabetes by diet and exercise alone and was instructed to start taking insulin injections once a day, before lunch. There was an option to take some pills, but the doctor felt it was necessary to move straight to insulin injections, based on my glucose chart mapping. I felt like a total failure and was quite upset at this. The endocrinologist reassured me that I had done nothing wrong and that some people simply can't control it through diet alone. I also have a history of diabetes in the family, since my dad and most of my uncles and aunts had it, so I was informed that I am also at a higher risk of developing full blown diabetes in the future. As each week passed, despite keeping my diet consistent, my insulin dosage amount had to be increased as my body was unable to cope. I eventually had to inject myself with insulin twice a day, and then subsequently three times a day, before each meal. At first, I hated the whole thought and motion of sticking a needle into my thigh. The first time, I closed my eyes and looked away before poking myself with the needle.

"I hateee this! I don't want to do it. It's going to suck." I was not a fan of needles.

I picked a random spot on my thigh and squeezed the insulin in with the needle. It didn't hurt at all.

"Huh." I said, pleasantly surprised. The needle point was so fine that it barely made a mark or caused any pain. "That wasn't so bad!"

For the most part, it became a routine part of my pregnant life. A couple of times it did hurt and bleed a little, but I managed to perfect pinpointing the spots where it wouldn't hurt. By the end of my pregnancy, it had almost become easier to stab myself with insulin that it was to try and maintain a strict diabetic diet and yet see the blood sugar levels rise dangerously. With the insulin, I was able to eat the same food and not see any noticeable spikes – my blood glucose levels were fairly stable when I checked them after my meals.

21

IT CAN BE POSSIBLE TO EXPERIENCE LOW BLOOD SUGAR LEVELS EVEN THOUGH YOU HAVE GESTATIONAL DIABETES.

At one point, for an entire week, I cut out all sugar from my diet. This, it turns out, is a really dangerous thing to do as well. My blood sugar levels dropped dangerously low - especially at night when I was eating less generally, since it was mostly snacks after 6pm according to my diet plan.

I nearly fainted at the hospital while waiting for an anatomy scan - I had woken up late and missed breakfast, then had a light lunch without any sugar - plain chicken and broccoli with a green tea. I have never fainted before in my life and it was a really scary feeling. My heart was pumping and I felt extremely light-headed and dizzy. My whole body was quivering and my vision got blurred, so I stood up suddenly, clutching the rails of the chair and looking quite pale, I assume. The other people in the waiting room looked at me curiously and I was mortified.

I am an introvert in every sense, and I felt like I was causing a scene as I said in a low voice "Arggh, I feel weird."

My mom, who was waiting with me, asked "Weird, how?" to which I replied, "I dunno, just weird, like all dizzy and stuff, and my heart is beating really fast. I think I'm going to faint!"

"Faint?!" she jumped out of her chair, as did my sister.

"I think so…? I've never fainted before… I don't know. I feel really light-headed and dizzy. I've never felt this way before."

"You haven't been eating properly! I told you!" my sister said anxiously, "I'm going to get you some food."

"I've been eating just fine," I snapped weakly, "I'm not hungry."

I sat back down as I felt like I was losing my balance. I was acutely aware of the people nearby looking at me. I wondered what they were thinking. Were they wondering if I was going to throw up on them? Maybe they were wondering what to do if I did faint. Or maybe they thought I was being overly dramatic. What would happen if I did faint? I'd hit the floor and hurt Little Fetus. *Yes, sitting down is a good idea*, I thought to myself. *How do you know if you're going to faint, if you've never fainted before?* Would I just slide off the chair and hit the floor anyway? I guess it would be easier to keep me in place if I fainted in a chair. The chair was really comfortable, I noted. At least the hospital kept in mind that pregnant ladies need comfy chairs in waiting rooms, I thought to myself.

My mom called out to the ultrasound department receptionist who simply looked at me and said, "You're pregnant, it's normal to feel like that." This made me feel quite annoyed, and so I frowned at her. I'm not sure if the frown actually reached my face, or if the thought of frowning just stayed in my head, since she didn't seem to notice. I was trying not to panic, as I felt more woozy. I was scared that Little Fetus might not get enough oxygen or something. I told her I had never felt like this before and she offered me a glass of water, which I accepted. My sister had run over to the nearby cafe and came back with a chicken sandwich and a bottle of apple juice, which I forced myself to eat despite not being hungry. It's hard to say no to your mom and sis sometimes. I was pleasantly surprised to find myself feeling better within five minutes as I chugged the apple juice and nibbled on the sandwich.

The receptionist came back to check on me with a cheery smile. When I said I was feeling fine, she nodded and said, "It is your turn for the scan, in about five minutes."

The scan went well, and it was noted that Little Fetus was going to be a very big baby as she was growing quite fast. It was possible that she could be 10 lbs if she went full term. My gestational diabetes was influencing her. Being a very small framed woman, it was quite possible that it would be difficult for Little Fetus to come out of me naturally.

Later that week, at a doctor's visit, I was told that cutting out all sugars was a bad move as the body needs some glucose to function. Low blood sugar levels were the reason for my symptoms - which I also had been experiencing nightly. She told me that drinking the apple juice was the best way of getting a quick shot of sugar in me fast and I was definitely able to agree to that. Gestational diabetes only lasts as long as the pregnancy lasts. I found this hard to believe, but it was true. The moment I gave birth to Little Fetus, I was told I could go back to eating and drinking normally as I had pre-pregnancy. I was skeptical, but immediately requested a Tim Horton's Iced Cappucino, which my husband already had anticipated and had waiting for me, along with a can of Pringles, and a bag of mini-twix bars.

- Pregnant women who have never had diabetes before but who end up having high blood glucose (sugar) levels during pregnancy are said to have gestational diabetes.
- Most pregnant women have a glucose screening test between 24 and 28 weeks of pregnancy. The test may be done earlier if you have a high glucose level in your urine during your routine prenatal visits, or if you have a high risk for diabetes
- Gestational diabetes is due to the mother's body being unable to make and use all the insulin it needs for pregnancy.
- Without enough insulin, glucose increases in the blood to high levels. This is called hyperglycemia
- Hormones from the pregnancy may be the reason

for some people developing gestational diabetes. The hormones may block the action of insulin in the mother's body. This is called insulin resistance. The mother may need as much as three times more insulin.

- Untreated or poorly controlled diabetes during pregnancy can harm your baby. The added sugars in the mother's blood travel to the baby through the placenta, causing the baby's blood glucose levels to rise. This causes the baby's pancreas to create more insulin. Since the baby is getting more energy than it needs, it is stored as fat and you can end up with a very large baby (macrosomia, or fat baby).
  - o Macrosomia can lead to a baby's shoulders being damaged during birth
  - o A very large baby may be unable to pass safely through the mother's birth canal, prompting a c-section
  - o Because of the extra insulin made by the baby's pancreas, newborns may have very low blood glucose levels at birth
  - o Macrosomia babies are at higher risk for breathing problems.
  - o Babies with excess insulin become children who are at risk for obesity and adults who are at risk for type 2 diabetes.
- Low blood sugar levels (hypoglycaemia) are more likely when a pregnant woman has gestational diabetes.
- In recent years it has become increasingly evident that insulin-dependent diabetic patients, whether pregnant or not, run a much increased risk of having severe hypoglycaemia attacks (i.e. the

patient needs the assistance of another person to relieve the attack) whenever attempts are made to introduce tight blood glucose control.

- Episodes of severe hypoglycaemia could have serious consequences.
    o It is especially hazardous for the mother particularly during the performance of a critical task such as driving a car.
    o Insulin-induced hypoglycaemia in the last trimester of diabetic pregnancy may increase fetal body movement and decrease the fetal heart rate variability.
    o A number of very rare conditions have been reported to be associated with severe hypoglycaemia, such as
        ▪ insulinoma
        ▪ severe malaria
        ▪ HELLP syndrome (haemolysis, elevated liver enzymes, low platelet count)
        ▪ severe fulminating liver disease
        ▪ ACTH and/or growth hormone deficiency

22

CHEESE IS AN EXCELLENT SOURCE OF PROTEIN, AND MAKES FOR A DELICIOUS DIABETIC LATE NIGHT SNACK WHEN PAIRED WITH CRACKERS.

Along with the insulin injections, I was instructed to pee on a small strip every morning right after I woke up and before I ate anything. This strip measured the keytones in my urine. The more keytones, the worse my diabetes management was. I also had to prick my finger six times a day with a needle to draw out a droplet of blood in order to check my blood sugar levels. Pricking my finger for this process hurt more than stabbing myself with a giant insulin needle. Sometimes, I'd prick my finger, but I wouldn't draw enough blood out, so I would have to prick myself again. I would have to touch the blood to a disposable test strip attached to a glucose meter which drew the blood in and measured the glucose levels in my blood. So of course, at other times, I would draw enough blood out, but then would somehow manage to not get enough of it on the test strip, so I'd have to prick myself again. I'd keep alternating fingertips just so an individual fingertip wouldn't get too tender.

Once before and after breakfast, lunch and dinner – six times a day, I'd write down the value shown in the glucose meter. I also had to track all the food I ate, the quantities I ate and the times I ate at. Writing all this down in a journal kept me on track in terms of managing my diet, but it also taught me so much about my dietary habits. When first diagnosed with gestational diabetes, I was sent to a nutrition class held at the hospital to learn about it and how to eat properly. There were about 4 other pregnant ladies there, all at varying stages of pregnancy. It was then that I realized how many carbs I ate daily and how unhealthy my food choices and combinations were. I was sent home with a giant chart of diet planning for the entire week, depicting combinations of food types and the amount of nutrition each provided. I could mix and match the items to reach my required thresholds for proteins, carbs, sugars etc. I also noticed how drastically my sugar levels were affected by the different foods I ate. Most surprising, I was astonished that a simple change in the brand of bread I ate caused a huge spike or decline in my blood sugar level. The most delicious option I could eat that caused my levels to remain stable were chicken shawarma wraps from a very specific eatery that my sister found for me. Just that one specific location. I tried to eat a shawarma from another location, but my sugar level shot up too high. The worst food for sugar spikes were white rice and potatoes. Protein never raised my blood sugar levels, so I happily ate a lot of meat with steamed vegetables. Cheese and crackers were also a great snack option I relished every night. Red "string hoppers" from a nearby south asian ethnic (tamil) food store were another option that allowed me to eat in abundance without causing much of a spike in my sugar levels – this was an excellent replacement for the usual white rice that I ate, because it was also quite filling so I wasn't left feeling hungry all day. Pastas were a huge no-no, and chocolates were unfortunately a no go as well, so I couldn't have any more hot chocolate drinks without guilt. My body was quite finicky about food it chose to react to.

23

ANATOMY SCANS CAN SHOW YOU MORE THAN JUST YOUR BABY'S GENDER.

The anatomy scan was something I waited for with great anxiety. Ever since I found out I was pregnant and had been drinking almost every night prior to that, I was terrified that I had harmed my unborn child somehow. I was so scared that the results would come back abnormal or that I would be told that the child could be born with a defect that I had caused. I was also terrified of any birth defects that happen when the mother does not ingest enough folic acid during the first trimester of the pregnancy. This was another area where I was left in anxious anticipation, since I had not been taking prenatal vitamins the first four weeks of my pregnancy. I was also not sure if my diet had been sufficient nutrition-wise for that time. I do have to say, however, that I had been craving a lot of the 'right' kinds of foods, despite not knowing that I was pregnant. I sincerely believe it it because my body already knew what was needed and sent signals trying to get me to eat healthier. I had craved broccoli and eggs more than usual. I also started having a serious craving for Cheerios and Cornflakes cereal. All very out of the ordinary for my eating habits. It was great that I had actually given into those cravings because I don't think my usual daily diet of rice and cookies would have been enough.

Folate Facts:

- Folate is a B vitamin (vitamin B9) that helps the body make new cells
- It is an essential nutrient found green, leafy vegetables, broccoli, peas, corn, oranges, grains, cereals, and meats.
- Folate is especially crucial for women who are pregnant or trying to get pregnant, because adequate intake can prevent major birth defects. This group should consume 400 to 800 mg of folic acid (the synthetic form of folate) a day o   Folic acid is used in multivitamins supplements because it is better absorbed
- Consuming folate/folic acid during the first few weeks of pregnancy, significantly and substantially lowers the risk of several different birth defects, including neural tube defects (NTDs).
  - The neural tube is the embryonic precursor to the brain and spinal column.
  - NTDs include very serious defects like spinal bifida and anencephaly, birth without part of the brain.
- Since the neural tube forms so early in pregnancy (day 26 to 28), folate deficiencies must be corrected before a woman knows

she is pregnant.

- o As a result, public health strategies mandate supplementation in food products: In both the United States and Canada, folic acid has been added to white flour since the late 1990's, where it finds its way into baked goods like bread. Following food fortification, neural tube defects have dropped.
- On the flip side, consuming excessive amounts of folic acid is also potentially dangerous. In recent years, studies have shown that excess folic acid during pregnancy may be tied to an increase in the baby's risk of developing an autism spectrum disorder. However, only an association was found, and not an actual causation
  - o In the study, mothers who had very high blood levels of folate at delivery were twice as likely to have a child with autism compared to mothers with normal folate levels.
  - o Researchers also found that mothers with excessive B12 levels were three times as likely to have a child with autism.
  - o The risk was greatest among mothers who had excess levels of both folate and B12 -- their risk was over 17 times that of a mother with normal levels of both nutrients, the investigators reported.

Spina Bifida and Down Syndrome are two common birth defects detected during the anatomy scan. Spina bifida is a type of birth defect called a neural tube defect. It occurs when the bones of the spine (vertebrae) don't form properly around part of the baby's spinal cord. The exact cause of this birth defect isn't known. Experts think that genes and the environment are part of the cause. For example, women who have had one child with spina bifida are more likely to have another child with the disease. Women who are obese or who have diabetes are also more likely to have a child with spina bifida. Spina bifida can be mild or severe. Most mild cases of spina bifida don't require treatment, apparently, and may not even be detected till later on in life when the person gets x-rayed for something unrelated.

Down syndrome is a congenital disorder caused by the presence of an extra 21st chromosome, also called trisomy 21. The scans do not give a definite answer as to whether a baby has Down syndrome, but it is used to help parents and clinicians decide whether further diagnostic tests are wanted. During the ultrasound, the tech measures the clear space in the folds of tissue behind a developing baby's neck. In babies with Down syndrome and other chromosomal abnormalities, fluid tends to accumulate here, making the space appear enlarged. "Increased nuchal translucency" refers to a measurement greater than 3 mm. This finding does not mean that the fetus actually has a chromosomal abnormality but tells you that the risks of some genetic disorders and birth defects, including Down syndrome, are increased. This measurement, taken together with the mother's age and the baby's gestational age, can be used to calculate the odds that the baby has Down syndrome. With nuchal translucency testing, Down syndrome is correctly detected in about 80% of cases. When performed with a maternal blood test, its accuracy may be improved.

Happily, the results came back fine for the baby's physical health. All ten fingers and ten toes were also accounted for. This should hopefully ease your mind a little if you were in similar shoes as I was.

- An anatomy ultrasound scan is usually scheduled for the 20th week of pregnancy
- It will be used to determine fetal anomalies, the baby's size, and weight
- It is used to measure growth ensuring the fetus is developing according to plan
- The ultrasound tech takes extensive measurements of many different anatomic parts of the fetus. The following parts are checked:
  - Face
  - Brain (ventricles, choroid plexus, mid-brain, posterior fossa, cerebellum, cisterna magna, measurements of anterior and posterior horns of lateral ventricles)
  - Skull (shape, integrity, BPD and HC measurements)
  - Neck (nuchal fold thickness)
  - Spine
  - Heart (rate, rhythm, 4-chamber views, outflow tract)
  - Thorax (shape, lungs, diaphragm)

- o Abdomen (stomach, kidneys, liver, bladder, wall, umbilicus, cord, abdominal circumference AC)
- o Limbs (femur, tibia, fibia, humerus, radius, ulna, hands, feet femur length FL)
- o Genitals (gender, abnormality)
- o Cervix (length and opening)
- Your baby's gender can be determined at this time, if positioned appropriately

My sister accompanied me to my 20th week ultrasound. I had to return for another ultrasound a few weeks later and both my mom and sister kept me company. It was a very joyful experience, and although I had already been to a few scans with my husband prior to this one, it was the first time I was able to see Little Fetus looking like an actual human baby, with clearly defined limbs and the most adorable nose. On the way to the appointment, my sister and I took numerous pictures and videos. She happily parked in the "Expectant Mothers" parking spot, but was unable to maneuver into it for some reason, so I got out from the passenger's side seat and switched to the driver's side, while she stood outside recording a video of us.

A car tried to pull in beside me and honked impatiently at me. They always talk about a mom's ferocious protective nature for their baby. They forgot to mention a sister's ferocious protective nature over their preggo sister. She cussed them out, shaking her fists angrily, "Didn't anyone ever tell you, you don't honk at a pregnant lady! Graaaaaah!!!!"

My mom thought it was hilarious and chuckled. They didn't notice her, unfortunately. Their car windows were all up and I guess it was pretty soundproofed. A family of four got out and cheerily waved at her as they passed by. She just stood shaking her head. I found it funny too, and laughed as I got down and waddled over to the building with my mom and sis.

As we were crossing from the car parking area to the entrance, my sister had waved her arms around as if shielding me, saying, "Pregnant lady coming through! Slow down, slow down!" to the embarrassment of both my mom and myself. By now, we should have been used to her antics, you'd think.

Preggo Brain happens, remember? Your memory is shot to crap and you'll stare blankly in response to even the simplest questions at the most inopportune times. The receptionist asked for my name and I just stood there, wondering what it was. My sister had to respond with my name and then the receptionist just ignored me for the rest of the time and directed all questions to her and my mom. I was mildly insulted and partially amused. I was also trying to remember how old I was and where I lived.

The anatomy scan was the longest I ever had, and it took almost an hour. We were waiting for much longer for other appointments to go by. We were five minutes late to our appointment and the receptionist tsk tsked us as she curtly said that someone else was taken ahead of us due to our tardiness. It was well worth the wait.

The ultrasound tech let us see the monitor for the most part, as she was taking all the measurements and screenshots. She spent quite a bit of time checking the heart chambers. It was fascinating watching the screen. She showed us the umbilical cord and the flashing images that depicted the blood pumping. She showed us the little tiny fingers and toes, the brain, the spine. I couldn't believe how much Little Fetus had grown since the last ultrasound several weeks ago. She let us watch as Little Fetus yawned and stretched inside of me - pointing out the nose and mouth as we were unfamiliar with deciphering the contents of the screen at first. Little Fetus was perfect, with no abnormalities detected. The tech was not allowed to tell us if she was healthy or not, as that was up to the doctor to review and then let us know, but she had a pretty good idea.

Instead, I asked, "If you were me, would you be worried?"

To which she responded, "No." with a big smile.

However, Little Fetus was most definitely a fat baby. "Look at those cheeks!" I said in awe, as I looked at one of the printouts showing her from the bottom of her chin facing upwards so we could see up her nose. I hoped I would be able to push her out without complications.

24

While it is not uncommon for pregnancy to cause low blood pressure, sometimes high blood pressure becomes a problem. Preeclampsia is a potentially serious problem during pregnancy. It sometimes develops without any symptoms. High blood pressure might develop slowly, but more commonly it has a sudden onset. At every visit to the doctor's office, they checked my blood pressure as an important part of prenatal care because the first sign of preeclampsia is commonly a rise in blood pressure.

When checking your blood pressure:

- A cuff is wrapped around your arm above your elbow and air is pumped into it
- The cuff inflates and briefly stops the blood flow in the main blood vessel in your arm. It will feel tight, but it shouldn't hurt.

- Then, the air in the cuff is slowly released. The cuff is attached to the monitor, which calculates your blood pressure and shows a reading to your midwife.
- The reading will show two figures that look like a fraction, for example, 110/70. The first, or top, number tells you your blood pressure as your heart pushes the blood round your body (systolic blood pressure). The second, or bottom, number is your blood pressure when your heart relaxes between beats (diastolic).
- Blood pressure that is 140/90 millimeters of mercury (mm Hg) or greater, documented on two occasions, at least four hours apart, is abnormal.
- Preeclampsia is a pregnancy complication characterized by high blood pressure and signs of damage to another organ system — usually after 20 weeks of pregnancy.
  - Left untreated, preeclampsia can lead to serious and even fatal complications for both mother and baby.
  - Previously, preeclampsia was only diagnosed if a pregnant woman had high blood pressure and protein in her urine. However, experts now know that it's possible to have preeclampsia, yet never have protein in the urine.
  - Other signs and symptoms of preeclampsia might include:

- Excess protein in your urine (proteinuria) or additional signs of kidney problems
- Severe headaches
- Changes in vision, including temporary loss of vision, blurred vision or light sensitivity
- Upper abdominal pain, usually under your ribs on the right side
- Nausea or vomiting
- Decreased urine output
- Decreased levels of platelets in your blood (thrombocytopenia)
- Impaired liver function
- Shortness of breath, caused by fluid in your lungs
- Sudden weight gain and swelling (edema) — particularly in your face and hands — often accompanies preeclampsia.

- But many of these things also occur in many normal pregnancies, so they're not considered reliable signs of preeclampsia.

If you do have high blood pressure, it is important to treat it. The risk of heart attack, stroke and other problems associated with high blood pressure doesn't go away during pregnancy. And high blood pressure can be dangerous for your baby, too. However, that being said, any medication you take during pregnancy can also affect your baby. Although some medications used to lower blood pressure are considered safe during pregnancy, others — such as angiotensin-converting enzyme (ACE) inhibitors, angiotensin receptor blockers (ARBs) and renin inhibitors — are generally avoided during pregnancy. Your healthcare provider will prescribe the proper medication and dosage.

I had to pee into a cup every visit. There's not much to be said for this. I never could easily pee on demand. Speaking of pee. By now, I had to pee almost every five minutes, it felt like. I used to be one of those people who could hold their pee all day - I would pee perhaps twice a day. By the end of my second trimester, I was practically running to the washroom the moment I got out of it. And sneezing. Oh gawd, no. To sneeze was to be in absolute fear of peeing. And let's not forget laughing out loud - which I tended to do quite often generally.

Peeing my pants in my mid-thirties was never something I had anticipated ever doing. Sometimes, laughing too much would result in an accidental pee. I said something mean to my husband one day, and he responded with "I hope you sneeze and pee." That really was a low blow, I thought. I couldn't help but giggle to myself, nonetheless.

Third Trimester

YOUR PREGNANCY WILL UNLEASH YOUR INSTINCTUAL ANIMAL WITHIN YOU.

Third trimester had me balloon out like a blimp. I was waddling everywhere and holding my back with one hand like a... pregnant lady. But I felt strangely energetic. I also had the sudden urge to clean and do random things around the house. This, apparently, is called 'nesting'. Nesting is the urge to clean and organize your home, which is supposedly in preparation of baby's arrival. I really was completely unaware that I was doing it until my husband, sister, mom and dad all had to lecture me on why it is a Very Bad Idea to use power tools like electric hedge saws while being 7 months pregnant. The bushes could be trimmed by any of a number of other people, but for some reason, I found myself trimming bushes outside.

My husband hid the power cord. My parents and sister

just hid the trimmer. That particular urge only lasted a couple of weeks, thankfully. I look back on it now and wonder what the heck I was thinking. I mean, sure, it was a light tool, but when I imagine everything that could have gone wrong, I can't help but want to kick myself, considering my balance was not entirely perfect at the time. But, I suppose it is hard arguing with a pregnant lady. Hiding stuff is just so much easier.

The constant cleaning didn't stop though. I even found myself steam cleaning the couches in the living room - something I had never (nor had anyone else) ever bothered to do before. I was vacuuming every day – I even vacuumed the dogs. The outdoor shoes were strewn all over the place in disarray in the closet on the main floor. I bought two shoe racks and organized everybody's shoes neatly in multiple rows, according to gender, colour and purpose. I pulled stray weeds from the garden using a claw-like device that didn't require any bending – it was not easy to use, but it certainly kept me busy.

.

26

YOU WILL LOVE BEING PREGNANT, EVEN WHEN
YOU FEEL TIRED AND ACHY AND TIRED AND ACHY.

At one point I had an appointment for something unrelated to my pregnancy where I had to wait for about half an hour with a bunch of other people in the waiting lobby. There were seats everywhere and plenty of space to sit, but of course, none of them were pregnant-lady friendly. There were downright torture to sit on and so I started walking around almost in circles. My sister was with me, following closely behind even though I told her I was fine. She was apprehensive at the thought of me suddenly fainting and falling, I think. Or maybe she was just worried that I'd somehow manage to get ahold of another power tool. It was an interesting wait, as suddenly everyone started talking to me as I waddled past them slowly.

"When are you due?"

"Oh man, you're gonna pop soon!"

"You having twins, hun?"

"Are you having a boy or a girl?"

"I remember being pregnant, it was easier to walk than sit sometimes too!"

I loved the attention. It was nice. I didn't notice it, but my sister said that practically everyone I walked by would be watching me with a "ooh, she's pregnant, how cute" look or whisper. Little kids are the best, they point at your belly and say "There's a baby in there!". Did I mention also I loved being pregnant, despite all the highs and lows and pains and aches? To think that a little innocent mini human being would be the result makes it all worthwhile. I constantly wondered what she would look like.

27

*SOME PEOPLE HAVE NO SENSE OF BOUNDARIES
AND PERSONAL SPACE AND WILL RUB YOUR BELLY
WITHOUT PERMISSION*

I think the most surprising thing about being pregnant was finding out that some people have no sense of respecting personal space when they see a pregnant body. Imagine you're out walking, minding your own business, not pregnant, and suddenly someone comes over and rubs your belly. They touch you without asking and don't back off when you look uncomfortable. People suddenly seem to think it is okay to do when you're pregnant. Some people at least had a little decency and asked me first if they could pat my belly, to which I would generally say "Okay" in a not very enthusiastic manner - so they would keep it short and that was great. Others would just grab my stomach and rub away like it was a lamp that a genie would pop out of. My parents and siblings were very respectful of my space, and I loved that. My husband had free reign to rub my belly all he wanted, since I didn't mind at all. But other relatives and friends, and even acquaintances, didn't quite understand my aversion to being touched.

Some women love it. I'm not one of those women.

I am the type of person who hasn't had a professional massage yet since I don't want to be touched by a stranger. (You can only imagine how exhausting and draining the whole birthing process was for me, right? I've never been poked and prodded by so many strangers in my entire life.) So yes, in general, people are extra friendly and courteous when you're pregnant. Some people aren't. But the majority are. It is a time in your life where you are spoiled by the ones who love you, (if it is your first child, anyway. I have no idea how it will be if I ever have another.) and it is a time in your life where you are given extra reverence, even by strangers, as a mother-to-be.

28

IF YOU HAVE A DOG, BEWARE.

"**E**EEEEEEEE!" The high-pitched little-girl scream startled me, as I was sitting in my car in a parking lot. The scream was actually by a man, looking quite red in the face and flustered.

"Stupid dog!" the man yelled at me, as he jumped into his car in embarrassment.

"I'm so sorry!" I tried to not laugh. "She's a sweetheart, really!"

He pulled out of the parking spot and drove away. I had been sitting in my car with Doggy in the backseat, with the windows rolled down a little. Hubby had popped into the grocery store to grab a few items quickly. The poor unsuspecting man had walked by to get into his car when she jumped up and smacked the inside of our car window with her paws, barking loudly and jumping around. It was so sudden that the man had squealed like a little girl in surprise and recoiled before turning around and spreading his hands flat against his car, as if under arrest. It was like he didn't know what had hit him.

After a moment, he turned back around, looking (and feeling, I'm quite sure) very foolish and embarrassed. She couldn't get to him since the windows were rolled up fairly high. *Hey, there's no shame in being scared by a suddenly barking and quite large dog.*

Once he had driven away, Doggy lay back down on the backseat in contentment, pleased with herself for having protected her mom from the Scary Short Man With Plastic Bag. I rolled up the window and put the air-conditioning on for the remainder of our wait.

Our dog wouldn't let people approach me during the later months of my pregnancy. She was fiercely protective and would growl and bark at strangers who tried to talk to me if I were walking her down the street. At home, she was a completely different dog - she'd follow me around the house calmly and loved to snuggle next to me. She was a puppy of about 5 months age when we first learned I was pregnant, and she grew quite large very quickly during my pregnancy. I was saddened that some people very vocally recommend giving up your dog if you have a baby on the way. I would inform these people that dogs are actually a great addition to the family, especially if you have a baby. I started with science - it is scientifically proven that dogs boost a baby's immune system. A protein in their dander has a preventive effect concerning asthma. Psychologically, there are numerous health benefits, as dogs lower stress in humans and provide companionship. Then I ended with my opinion - dogs are simply the best. They provide unconditional love and loyalty and are a fantastic and beneficial member of your family if you provide them with the right training and care. Your dog has no malice or bad intentions - dogs just want a neck or back scratch and some food and they are as happy as can be. Throw in some walks and playtime and you've got the most loyal and devoted companion you could ever hope for. When you're pregnant and wondering if that sound outside is a burglar or just a bunny, your dog will be a source of comfort. When your baby comes along, that baby has a furry companion that will boost your little one's development and immune system.

- A study found that children's risk for developing allergies and asthma is reduced when they are exposed in early infancy to a dog in the household.
    - The study, funded by the National Institute of Allergy and Infectious Diseases (NIAID), is published online in the Proceedings of the National Academy of Sciences (PNAS) and involves a multi-disciplinary group of researchers from UCSF, the University of Michigan, Henry Ford Health System and Georgia Regents University.
- Psychologists at Oregon State University found that teaching children to care for a puppy enhanced their social skills, teaching them to be more cooperative and generous regarding sharing
- In another study, children who were regularly

given the opportunity to care for a puppy at their preschool, and those with pets at home were found to be more socially competent. They were more popular, felt better about themselves and were better able to understand other children's feeling

- Various studies have shown that having a dog in the household actually increases their owner's life span over time due to the cumulative positive effect of having a dog.

29

The other sad reality is that, sometimes, your pregnancy will make other people sad. Those who are suffering with infertility or who have suffered miscarriages. Those who are still waiting for Mr. or Mrs. Right to come along and don't feel like adoption is an option. Those who have to think about freezing their eggs and those who desperately want children but just can't, for whatever reason. Some of them will tell you outright how they feel, and it will break your heart because you know you are a reminder of something that breaks their heart. I had one person come right up to me and admit that my pregnancy made her feel sad. That being said, it made me feel a little guilty when I was around her, but I appreciated her honesty.

You question, why not them? You know they're questioning, why her and not me? I understood it, so it didn't make me feel too upset when I knew someone wasn't able to fully rejoice in my pregnancy or failed to be sympathetic to my complaints. When I hit 30 and Mr. Right was nowhere in sight, I wondered why I was unable to find someone who would be a good father to our future child. I resolved to either adopt or get a sperm donor if I didn't meet anyone within the next five years. There is still a cultural taboo around these options. I wish that wasn't the case.

I was also told by the doctor that at age 35, if I were to get pregnant, I would be considered a high-risk pregnancy. I was 34 when I gave birth to Little Fetus. This was not something that I needed to hear, nor did I feel it was warranted. A few relatives of mine had their first kid in their early to mid-forties. They weren't able to have more kids, but they did manage to have at least one. It creates a lot of pressure and sadness when these things are said to us as women. You never hear a man being told, you're getting old, you better have kids soon. There's this misconception that only women have to fear aging, because men can produce sperm throughout their lives. However, what they (whoever "they" are... society at large, perhaps?) forget to tell you is that there is a growing body of evidence that proves that the risks for men fathering children late in life are also significant. Research suggests that middle-aged men might be more likely to father children with mental health problems, as well as rare genetic disorders, such as the most common type of dwarfism. There is an increased risk of epilepsy, autism and breast cancer in their offspring.

Although men can produce sperm throughout their lives, the quality of that sperm does decline with age.

- Worldwide data from more than 60 teams of researchers on the health risks associated with older fathers found that men aged over 35 had a 50 per cent lower chance of conceiving over a 12-month period than younger men, even after taking into account the age of the would-be mother.
- The risk of miscarriage and premature birth also rises when the man is more than 40. A study of 23,821 pregnant women analysed by the researchers found that pregnancies involving men aged 50 or older were twice as likely to end in the loss of the foetus compared to younger fathers.
- Children conceived by fathers over 40 also have
  - a 30 per cent increased risk of epilepsy
  - a 37 per cent higher risk of Down's syndrome
  - a 14 per cent greater chance of childhood leukaemia, and
  - a 70 per cent greater likelihood of central nervous system cancers (such as brain tumours).
- If the father is over 45, there is a threefold increased risk of retinoblastoma, a rare type of eye cancer.
- Older fathers are thought to be at higher risk of having children with autism and schizophrenia.

So why do they make it seem like all the pressure should only be on women? I know plenty of older couples who have had kids without any problems. Sometimes things go wrong, and there's no explanation as to why. Sometimes things go well, and there's no explanation why. But you're thankful. Or oblivious. The topic is a complicated one. You have druggies popping out unwanted babies at all ages, abandoning them or worse. And then you have a friend who you know would absolutely be the best parent on the planet but was unable to become a mom or dad for reasons out of their control. And you wonder, why not them? Life doesn't make sense. And life isn't always fair. That's a fact.

There are women who have had far worse pregnancies than I have had - I know friends who had to be put on bed-rest, or who had to worry over abnormal results during their tests.

One lady reproached me sternly when I complained about hating being pregnant – "Be thankful. You are blessed. Do you know how many women would love to be in your position? Don't complain. Be grateful."

I was very taken aback, as I had not meant it in that way at all. I didn't mean that I hated being pregnant – I meant more that the pregnancy symptoms weren't something I was thrilled about. But upon reflection, I knew what she meant. There are many women out there who have no sympathy for your complaints, and most times these are women who have had experienced difficulties with their own pregnancy journey.

I am not saying that mine was terrible, but only that it was not exactly pleasant. All I ever heard from the people immediately around me was how easy their pregnancies were and how their babies just popped right out. I never heard any details concerning the weird hair growth, extra flatulence, aches, pains or worries. But I read somewhere that we are programmed to forget the whole pregnancy once the baby is born - our bodies are flooded with the appropriate hormones or processes that ensure we will not be averse to getting pregnant again and propagating the human species. This is entirely true, I believe, because nobody could remember most of their pregnancy details other than a general overview. I barely remember mine now, and it is only because I kept a rough written journal and an extensive video journal that I remember half as much as I do.

Anyway, my point is that I think sometimes we are not allowed to complain about our pregnancies because we are supposed to be grateful to have become pregnant in the first place. I can only hope that I do not offend anyone, but I think it is also important to share all the little details that nobody expects out of a normal pregnancy and to be allowed to say that some parts were uncomfortable or undesirable. If our pain or discomfort is not the worst pain that can be felt, it does not lessen the pain that we feel in that moment and should not preclude us from expressing those feelings appropriately. Just make sure you find a sympathetic ear and it is probably best to be empathetic - if you know someone has experienced worse, find someone else instead of discussing your complaints with them.

By the time I hit the last month of my pregnancy, I lost a lot of that initial energy. Some days, I could barely get out of bed. As I grew larger and larger, I found it harder to walk and even harder to just turn around and shift position while sleeping. It took me an entire minute or two to turn from my left side to my right side while sleeping. Hubby would have to help me get out of bed some mornings. My belly grew enormously large, even though the rest of me didn't really get fatter by a whole lot.

I started to have horrible shooting pains throughout my lower back that would even reach all the way to my lower calves. After a visit to the doctor I was assured that these were just normal third trimester pains.

If I dropped anything on the floor, it was almost comical as I tried to pick it up. I perfected the art of using my toes as fingers.

"That's disgusting! Monkey toes!" my sister gaped, shocked as I picked up a fallen piece of paper with my toes and handed it to myself.

"Hey, you wish you had toes like these!" I said, as I picked up a dog toy with my toes and tried to fling it at her.

"Stop, eww! That's so not normal!" she ran off to tell my dad about what she had just witnessed.

Around this time, Hubby and I decided to have a professional maternity photoshoot done. It was hilarious at points, as the photographer made us change into various outfits and use fun props. At one point both Hubby and I were almost topless, and I was leaning towards a fan, my body covered with a thin cloth, while Hubby stood behind me with his arms around me, trying to spit my 'wind-swept' hair out of his mouth. I tried to stop it from flying into my own eyes. Those photos have not seen the light of day, but they are a funny memory we three share – yes, my sister was a witness to these photos being taken, so we can't deny they exist. A lot of the photos did come out quite beautifully and I will cherish them till the end of my days. I noted that they edited out the linea nigra and all of the stretch marks and general discolorations caused by my pregnancy. If you're thinking about doing it – do it!

30

I got up one day in the middle of the night, and walked to my sister's room.

"What's up?" she asked, sitting up. I burst into tears at the foot of her bed. All I could say was "I'm so itchy. I can't take it anymore".

"Let's call your doctor first thing in the morning and set you up with an appointment." she suggested. She knew I hated going to the doctor and being poked and prodded, so she wasn't sure if I would agree.

"I think you're right. I just can't deal with this anymore. It's getting worse. It's been almost three weeks of this and I can't take it anymore." I sobbed.

This was the absolute worst part of my pregnancy - it was an almost unbearable itchy hive-like rash that suddenly appeared during the last three weeks of my pregnancy. It wasn't so bad when it started, but progressively got worse. It started as a small itchy red area on my waist, at the left side. As I itched, it got bumpier and wider. Within a week, it covered my entire belly and sides. My skin was tearing from the itching and it became inflamed and looked horrifying as the skin tore and bled. The more I itched, the worse it got. It was almost impossible to try not itching because it was a constant, unrelenting feeling. It just wouldn't stop feeling itchy.

The next morning, bright and early, we went to the doctor's office and a resident checked me over. She prescribed an ointment and sent me home. The rash just got worse. I went back three days later and was seen by an older, much more experienced doctor. She prescribed a different cream that contained a custom made mix of herbal and cortisol ingredients. She also sent me to get my blood tested for possible liver problems as sometimes the liver is affected during pregnancy and a rash was a symptom of liver failure during pregnancy. When the tests came back negative, she then sent me to a specialist ob/gyn to be seen for the remainder of my pregnancy as she felt I needed to be looked after more closely. She diagnosed me with "PUPPP".

- Pruritic urticarial papules and plaques of pregnancy (PUPPP) is a hives-like rash that strikes some women during pregnancy.
- The exact cause of the skin condition is

unknown, but certain studies suggest fetal cells migrate to the mother's skin, causing inflammation.

- It is extremely itchy and causes major discomfort to the mother-to-be, but isn't dangerous to the fetus.
- It stops almost immediately after giving birth.

31

SOMETIMES EXTREME ITCHINESS CAN BE A SIGN OF CHOLESTASIS, WHICH CAN BE FATAL FOR YOUR FETUS.

If your palms and feet are itchy, or even other parts of your body, mention it to your doctor. This itchiness can occur earlier, but it generally begins during the later weeks of the third trimester. A simple blood test can rule out cholestasis - which refers to any condition that impairs the flow of bile — a digestive fluid — from the liver. Pregnancy can be a cause of cholestasis.

32

The ointments and creams that the doctors gave me didn't help at all. I googled all night and came up with a recommendation from several other moms-to-be on a few online forums - pine tar soap. It was available for cheap at the local Bulk Barn. It works, people! It works!

I kid you not - it worked almost immediately. I stood in the shower, closing my eyes in hopeful anticipation as I rubbed a foamy thick lather of the soap suds all over my itchy belly. Now for the result - I stepped out of the shower and toweled myself off. Showers generally were all I had to keep me sane, they stopped the itching temporarily, and for at least 20 minutes after I stepped out of the shower. However, it is not practically possible to have 15 showers a day. After this particular shower, two hours passed and I was still not itching. I couldn't believe it. Yay! I was giddy with happiness. From then on, I was able to get by on 3 showers a day to ease the itch. The bumps even went down and turned from reddish pink to a deeper brown. The wounds healed. The PUPPP rash left my skin scarred for months - but I generally scar easily and it takes a long time for my skin to go back to normal.

33

IF YOUR BELLY IS LARGER THAN MOST, YOU MAY HAVE EXCESS AMOUNTS OF AMNIOTIC FLUID

The specialist I was referred to was extremely attentive. He checked my belly, looked at my diabetes chart and medical history, asked me a few questions, and then suggested that we schedule a c-section as soon as possible. He said I also had an excessive amount of amniotic fluid - something that only 1 percent of pregnant women get, apparently. Yay, me.

I was at 37 weeks when we saw the specialist. He stated that the baby would potentially be in danger if she were to go past 39 weeks and wanted to schedule the c-section at the beginning of week 38. My husband and I pondered about this for a while, and I knew from a little research that women who have gestational diabetes have a higher risk of a stillbirth. This, of course, was something I absolutely didn't want to risk. There was also a higher risk of spontaneous abortion and preeclampsia. However, I also knew that babies being born prematurely can have complications, such as their lungs not being matured enough. I was unsure if it was the right option, but decided to wait till the end of week 38. I wanted to elect to have the c-section, but my husband gently convinced me to try for a natural birth first through induction - another option that the specialist had presented us with. I had never had any surgeries before and c-sections came with their own set of risks for the mother. Even my endocrinologist had told me earlier that most doctors generally don't recommend c-sections if it can be helped. Little Fetus wasn't due for another few weeks and we figured we would give her all the time we could spare for her to continue developing.

I agreed to be induced the following Monday, at the end of my 38th week of her gestation.

- Polyhydramnios (pol-e-hy-DRAM-nee-os) is the excessive accumulation of amniotic fluid — the fluid that surrounds the baby in the uterus during pregnancy. Polyhydramnios occurs in about 1 percent of pregnancies.
- Severe polyhydramnios may cause:
  - shortness of breath
  - preterm labor
  - Premature rupture of membranes — when your water breaks early
  - Excess fetal growth
  - Placental abruption — when the

placenta peels away from the inner wall of the uterus before delivery

- o Umbilical cord prolapse — when the umbilical cord drops into the vagina ahead of the baby
- o C-section delivery
- o Stillbirth
- o Heavy bleeding due to lack of uterine muscle tone after delivery

- Mild polyhydramnios may go away on its own. Severe polyhydramnios may require treatment, such as draining the excess amniotic fluid.
- The earlier that polyhydramnios occurs in pregnancy and the greater the amount of excess amniotic fluid, the higher the risk of complications.

34

IT IS POSSIBLE TO BE HAVING CONTRACTIONS AND TO NOT KNOW IT.

The specialist sent me to the hospital to have some tests done to make sure that Little Fetus was doing fine, including "electronic fetal heart monitoring" and a "nonstress test". The tech hooked me up to some things and left me in a room for a while. Little lines went up and down on the monitor. My sister and I looked at each other a little apprehensively, wondering why exactly I had been sent for this.

The tech returned periodically. Finally, I was all done and she said, "Everything looks great! She's a happy baby! She's a very active baby. I've never seen such an active baby before."

"That's what everyone keeps telling me." I said, patting my belly and immediately feeling and seeing Little Fetus kick me back as I pulled my shirt back over my belly.

My entire belly wobbled.

"What do contractions feel like?" I asked her, for no particular reason, and out of the blue.

The tech looked at me in mild puzzlement as she asked, "Don't you feel those contractions?"

I looked at her blankly, "What contractions?"

"You're having mild contractions. Lots of them." She said with a smile. "Your little one is ready to come out anytime now. I'd even say by the end of the week."

"But I can't feel anything!" I exclaimed in surprise.

"It happens," she replied with a reassuring smile, "Don't worry, as long your baby is fine it is nothing to worry about. And she's doing more than fine."

I left, perplexed. *It happens? Nobody told me it happens.* I did some research and yes, there is such a thing as "silent contractions" and even "silent labor" where the woman can't feel the contractions and some do not experience labor pains. *If I can't feel any contractions, how will I know when I am in active labor?* I pondered.

- Electronic fetal heart monitoring is done during pregnancy, labor, and delivery. o It keeps track of the heart rate of your fetus.
    - o It also checks the duration of the contractions of your uterus.

[137]

- Your baby's heart rate is a good way to tell if your baby is doing well or may have some problems.
- External monitoring is used for a nonstress test. This test records your baby's heart rate while your baby is moving and not moving.
- A nonstress test may be done with a fetal ultrasound to check the amount of amniotic fluid.
- External monitoring is also done for a contraction stress test. This test records changes in your baby's heart rate when you have contractions.
    o It may be done to check on your baby's health if your baby does not move enough during a nonstress test.
    o It may help predict whether your baby can handle the stress of labor and vaginal delivery.

35

THERE'S AN OLD WIVES TALE THAT FULL MOONS CAN CAUSE EARLY LABOR.

That following weekend, on the Saturday, there was a beautiful full moon. There was also a total lunar eclipse. It was both a "supermoon" or a "bloodmoon" and it was a rare "total eclipse of a supermoon". Wow. I vaguely remembered reading stuff in the past about animals giving birth more on full moon days, statistically. I had also heard an old wives tale about humans giving birth more on full moon days. I wondered if Little Fetus would decide to pop out early. *Nah.* It was too early, and those are just stupid stories.

Yeah, you guessed it - Little Fetus decided she wanted to try and come out early. It was the weekend of the full moon when I went into early labor, on the Saturday.

"I think I'm having contractions," I woke Hubby up.

[139]

"You are?! Should we head to the hospital?" He was already changing into his jeans.

"I'm not sure," I said, feeling waves of pain at random intervals. The pain was significant enough for me to not dismiss them. "Let's just wait till they're more consistent in timing, they're really irregular right now."

"Alright," he was looking around for the little suitcase he had packed for us for an overnight stay at the hospital.

A cousin of mine had sent a very detailed list of items we might have wanted to consider packing. I honestly have no idea what Hubby ended up packing for us, but I do remember that he had thought of almost everything, including the infant car seat. My sister brought the items he had not thought of, such as the lotions, creams, toothpaste, etc. My mom bought the ridiculously priced, yet safe and dependable, Britax baby stroller. There was nothing I had to do or think of, it had all been done and thought of for me, and I know how lucky I am that this was the case.

Here's the list of items my cousin had suggested, in case you find it helpful:

THE ULTIMATE HOSPITAL BAG CHECKLIST

- **FOR JOURNEY TO HOSPITAL**
  - o Inco pad or old towel
  - o Black bag

- **FOR ME IN LABOUR**
  - o Dressing robe
  - o Flip flops for shower
  - o Slippers to walk around in?
  - o Fuzzy pink socks with rubber on the bottom
  - o Massage oils or lotions and tennis ball/wooden thingy
  - o Lip balm
  - o Headphones
  - o Hairband and hair clips
  - o Bendy straws
  - o Water spray (evian in fridge)
  - o Hand held fan
  - o My phone & charger
  - o St Thomas' orange maternity book
  - o Contact lenses and glasses
  - o Snacks – Chocolate, cookies, dates, jelly
  - o Small packs of coconut water and capri sun
  - o Magazines
  - o Maternity body pillow for breastfeeding

- **FOR HUBBY**
  - o A change of clothes and chuddies/vest/socks
  - o Warm puffalump Jumper

- o mini cologne/deodorant
- o Eyemask and earplugs
- o Towel
- o Shower flipflops
- o PJs/Scrubs
- o Cash for snacks in hospital
- o iPad, movies, magazines
- o Music playlist
- o Pillow
- o Camera or camcorder and charger
- o Paracetamol just in case!
- o Comfortable shoes – you might be pacing the corridors!
- o Phone & phone charger
- o Headphones
- o Snacks and drinks for yourself
- o Toothbrush/toothpaste

- **FOR ME POSTPARTUM**
  - o Going-home blue stripe dress (loose comfy clothes, no low waistbands) & flatties
  - o Primark 2 nightdresses (front opening for breastfeeding)
  - o Warm puffalump Jumper
  - o Few changes of clothes in case you stay a few days in hospital
  - o Nursing bras x2-3
  - o Crappy panties (big high waisted ones for LSCS)
  - o Breastfeeding info leaflets
  - o Breast pads (for leakages)
  - o Nipple cream lansinoh
  - o Maternity pads (x24)

- o Toiletries – deodorant, travel sized shampoo/conditioner/shower gel
- o Make up remover cream and face pads
- o Towel
- o Shower cap
- o Ear plugs (in case you end up on a noisy ward) and eyemask
- o Tissues
- o Wet wipes
- o Plastic bags for dirty laundry
- o 1 roll of soft toilet paper in case I have stitches
- o Wesley
- o Comb, hairdryer, GHDs
- o Toothbrush and toothpaste
- o Lipstick, powder, blusher, mirror, eyeliner, face moisturiser, perfume

- **FOR BABY:**
  - o 6x sleepsuits (with feet and scratch mits) – newborn size & 0-3mth size
  - o 6x vests
  - o 1x cardigan
  - o One outfit for the trip home. All-in-one stretchy outfits are best
  - o Baby blanket
  - o Hat
  - o Newborn nappies (may need up to 12 per day!!)
  - o Muslin squares
  - o Cotton wool
  - o Nail care kit
  - o Vaseline

- o 6 x bibs
- o Infant car seat – REAR FACING

- **KEEP IN CAR:**
  - o Spare sleepsuits
  - o spare duffel bag for extra stuff eg pressies

We rushed to the hospital in the dead of the night as my contractions got more painful. *I guess I didn't have to worry about not being able to tell.*

I was sent home, though, because after an entire day of waiting in the hospital, 8 hours later, the labor symptoms suddenly stopped.

36

LABOR CAN STOP.

I looked at the doctor in disbelief. "What do you mean? Is the baby okay? How can it just stop? Nobody told me it can just stop?!"

My husband and I looked at each other in confusion. Pregnant ladies were waddling and heaving all around me in the labour waiting room. One very pregnant lady was extremely irritable, as she kept slamming her hands on various desks and yelling, "Get this baby out of me!!!!" Another lady was being wheeled out, newborn in hand, big smile on her face, surrounded by aaaaahs and oooohs from the people around her.

"Well, you said you don't have any more labor pains or symptoms. Don't worry. It happens sometimes. If you don't feel like being induced, you can go home. Come back when you feel contractions again."

Apparently, there were LOTS of babies being born that day. More than usual. Go figure.

"It's all the winter babies!" a nurse cheerily explained. "People get extra frisky during December, it seems."

They had checked me and found that I was indeed in active labor - dilated a few centimeters. I had also bled a bit, and was told that this is normal. I had lost my mucus plug a few days earlier which was also normal. (A mucus plug is quite disgusting if you catch a glimpse of it while on the toilet. It's like a giant red-green snott ball that doesn't come out of your nose, but out of your hoo-ha instead. Throughout your pregnancy, the mucus plug blocks the opening of the cervix to prevent bacteria from entering the uterus. A short time before labor, this mucus plug is expelled, (the time before it is discharged differs for each woman, and some women don't even realize or notice it when it is is expelled) allowing the baby to pass through the cervix during labor and birth.

I was offered the option to be put on induction fluids. I opted to wait till Monday, since I was already scheduled for the induction at that point. So, technically, I was in active labour for two days, albeit without much symptoms. It was weird and I was completely unprepared for it.

Monday came, and I was given induction fluids. My water was not breaking, so the doctor had to manually break it. So much liquid poured out of me, I thought it would never stop. I opted to have the epidural, as the contractions pain got worse.

"It is normal to feel itchy after this. It's a side effect of the drugs." the anesthesiologist said to me as he poked something into my lower spine area.

"So that's why all the druggies in the movies always scratch themselves! I'd always wondered about that." it was truly a revelation for me.

He seemed amused by this and tried to hide a smile.

I was unable to push Little Fetus out, try as I might. During most of my labor, the baby's heartrate was strong and steady. Then, it started slowing at times. Every time it slowed to a certain point, the nurse would come in and shift my body around until the baby's heart rate became steady again. She stated that the loss of amniotic fluid was causing the baby's umbilical cord to get compressed more easily since there was no liquid cushioning. This was causing the baby's heart rate to slow as her oxygen and blood supply became interrupted. I tried my hardest not to move too much, which was difficult each time I tried to push her out. As my contractions continued, I started feeling weaker and weaker for some reason and felt really sleepy, almost like I was passing out. At around 11pm, when the slowing of her baby's heartbeat became more frequent, they hooked something directly to the baby in order to monitor her heart rate and to make sure that it wasn't my own heartbeat that was slowing down.

At midnight exactly, her heart actually stopped.

It started again after a few seconds of skipping some beats. The nurse paged the doctor right away.

I was sobbing when the doctor came in and she said what I already knew. I was feeling like my baby was in danger and wondering why they weren't just getting her out of me. Apparently, every other mother-to-be was having a c-section that day. "I think we need to do an emergency c-section. I was hoping you, at least, wouldn't need one. But it looks like she is starting to get sick so we need to move quickly."

The c-section experience was not pleasant mostly due to the sense of urgency and the tension that was almost tangible and palpable to me, even though all the medical staff kept their voices light and casual. I was wheeled to the surgery room, and my body was lifted onto the operating bed. My hands were then outstretched on either side of my body and strapped down. They put more drugs into me. Hubby was finally let in and he came and sat beside my head, wide eyed and serious. I had to ask him to lighten up and tell me some jokes because he was starting to freak me out. A curtain of sorts was raised in front of me so I couldn't see them operating on me, but Hubby had a good view of what was going on. The room was full of doctors, nurses and the anesthesiologist within minutes of me being laid on the table and strapped down. I was told that my endocrinologist and a neonatologist (newborn pediatric specialist) were also present. Halfway through the surgery, the drugs sent my body into a crazy shaking mode. I was shivering without being cold. I don't remember exactly how much time went by, but I was surprised at how quickly they took our little one out. I felt a strong sense of pressure and then heard her little cry. It was overwhelmingly wonderful to hear her cry. They let me kiss her but I was unable to hold her as I was still being operated on - it took a whole lot longer for them to stitch me back up. I had lost quite a bit of blood and was monitored closely afterwards as they were undecided whether I would need a blood transfusion. A form had been required to be filled out when I first got to the hospital asking for information and preferences. I had indicated on my preferences that I was unsure if I would like a blood transfusion, so they were taking that preference into account.

"You're young and healthy, your body will most likely cope, but we are monitoring you. You were borderline transfusion level." the nurse said as she wheeled me into a private room to rest after the surgery. I was blissfully holding my baby to my chest, so I didn't think to ask any questions about it.

37

A beautiful little baby was born. And while this was the end of my pregnancy story, it was also the start of her story. I wished all the blessings and happiness upon her the moment I got to hold her in my arms. And I wish the same for you and your little one(s).

Made in the USA
Lexington, KY
06 May 2017